# The Guide to Medical Staff Bylaws

Mary J. Hoppa, MD, MBA

HCPro

*The Guide to Medical Staff Bylaws* is published by HCPro, a division of BLR.

 5 4 3 2 1

Download the additional materials of this book at *www.hcpro.com/downloads/11777*.

ISBN: 978-1-61569-293-4



HCPro provides information resources for the healthcare industry.

HCPro is not affiliated in any way with The Joint Commission, which owns the JCAHO and Joint Commission trademarks.

Mary J. Hoppa, MD, MBA, Author
Karen Kondilis, Editor
Adam Carroll, Proofreader
Adrienne Trivers, Product Manager
Erin Callahan, Senior Director, Product
Shane Katz, Cover Image

Advice given is general. Readers should consult professional counsel for specific legal, ethical, or clinical questions.

Arrangements can be made for quantity discounts. For more information, contact:

HCPro
75 Sylvan Street, Suite A-101
Danvers, MA 01923
Telephone: 800-650-6787 or 781-639-1872
Fax: 800-639-8511
Email: *customerservice@hcpro.com*

**Visit HCPro online at *www.hcpro.com* and *www.hcmarketplace.com***

2/2014

# Contents



  

# About the Author

## Mary J. Hoppa, MD, MBA

Mary J. Hoppa is a senior consultant with The Greeley Company, Inc., in Danvers, Mass. She brings more than 25 years of healthcare leadership and management experience to her work with physicians, hospitals, and healthcare organizations across the country. Dr. Hoppa's roles in hospital administration and medical staff leadership in academic and community hospital settings make her uniquely qualified to assist physicians and medical centers in developing effective solutions to their most significant challenges. She has experience in credentialing and privileging, peer review and quality, medical staff education, and conflict resolution, and is the leader of The Greeley Company's bylaws division. She brings this experience into the accreditation practice.

Dr. Hoppa is one of The Greeley Company's leading national speakers and is the author or coauthor of the following HCPro/Greeley books: *The Top 40 Medical Staff Policies and Procedures,* Fourth Edition (2010); *The Medical Executive Committee Handbook,* Third Edition (2007); and *The Medical Staff Leaders' Practical Guide,* Sixth Edition (2007). Dr. Hoppa is a family physician with 15 years of post-residency practice experience, including chief medical officer at Methodist Hospital in Merrillville, Ind. Dr. Hoppa's previous positions include physician advisor, medical director of an employed physician group, medical director of various insurance plans, and member of the Iowa Board of Medical Examiners.

Dr. Hoppa is a graduate of the University of Wisconsin Medical School and School of Business. She received her residency training at the Mercy/St. Luke's Family Practice Residency Program in Davenport, Iowa.

# How to Use This Book

Organized medical staffs are an established feature of the hospital landscape in the United States. The maintenance of a medical staff is necessary if a hospital wishes to participate in federal health reimbursement programs and seek accreditation. Furthermore, the Centers for Medicare & Medicaid Services' *Conditions of Participation* require each medical staff to have written bylaws, and this requirement is echoed in the standards of accrediting bodies such as The Joint Commission (TJC), Det Norske Veritas (DNV), the Healthcare Facilities Accreditation Program of the American Osteopathic Association (HFAP), and the Center for Improvement in Healthcare Quality (CIHQ).

This book is intended to help medical staffs that want to review their current bylaws documents and determine whether change is warranted. A complete model set of bylaws is not provided because each medical staff's bylaws must mirror the uniqueness of the medical staff for which it is written. The saying "form follows function" applies here. Once a medical staff decides how it wants to function, those decisions should be incorporated into its medical staff bylaws.

As you read through the sections that follow, you will see that various medical staff design options are outlined for the reader's consideration. This book provides examples of bylaws language that illustrate various approaches to medical staff governance, organizational structure, and process.

However, it is important that medical staffs do not simply copy and paste this sample language word for word in their own bylaws, as it may need to be tailored to accommodate varying circumstances. Always seek legal counsel before making any revisions to your bylaws language. The careless adoption of sample medical staff bylaws language is a practice that can get an institution into trouble.

Because this book is divided into sections that reflect bylaws issues that medical staffs most commonly struggle with, it can be read either as a comprehensive orientation to a bylaws redesign or in a targeted manner as medical staff leaders ponder specific issues. It is recommended that a medical staff governance task force look carefully at all aspects of the organization's functions at least once every three years to gauge whether changes to the bylaws would be prudent. In the interim, this book also serves as a resource for incremental changes to bylaws when circumstances warrant them.

Every effort has been made to ensure that the book's content is current as of its publication date. Much of what is written is influenced and constrained by current federal and state regulations, court rulings, and accreditation standards. Because these are subject to frequent change, readers should always carefully review the latest version of accreditation standards and seek knowledgeable counsel before adopting changes to their existing bylaws.

The terminology used in the sample bylaws language may differ from that used at your institution. In most cases, it will be clear where logical substitutions can be made. For example, "trustee" may be used in place of "director;" "chief of staff" may replace "president of the medical staff;" "vice president of medical affairs" may be substituted for "chief medical officer;" and so forth. All percentages, numbers, and timelines in the sample bylaws language are for demonstration purposes only and should be altered to reflect the preferences at your institution.

This book was written with one of Albert Einstein's quotes in mind: "All things should be made as simple as possible, but not simpler." In suggesting medical staff design possibilities, always try to look for ways to reduce bureaucracy that does not add value, and add approaches that create a more streamlined organization. Sometimes less can be more.

This book is organized into six major sections. Section 1 addresses preliminary information, such as the bylaws' table of contents, preamble, and definitions. Section 2 tackles issues of medical staff governance and structure, such as staff categories; the difference between membership and privileges; membership responsibilities and rights; officers; medical executive committee composition; and amending the bylaws. Section 3 focuses on collegial intervention, investigations, corrective action, and fair hearings. Section 4 delves into issues related to credentialing and privileging, including focused professional practice evaluation, ongoing professional practice evaluation, and the aging practitioner. Section 5 addresses the issues of credentialing and the fair hearing and appeal process for advanced practice professionals. Section 6 concludes with various operational issues, such as determining the appropriate number of committees, introducing a new committee for medical staff leadership and succession planning, and setting quorum and attendance requirements.

I hope the organization of this book helps to focus your attention where it matters most.

—Mary J. Hoppa, MD, MBA

# DOWNLOAD YOUR MATERIALS NOW

To access the sample bylaws language in this book, please visit the website listed below. Please note that this sample bylaws language is not appropriate in every circumstance, is not complete, and is not provided as legal advice.

**www.hcpro.com/downloads/11777**

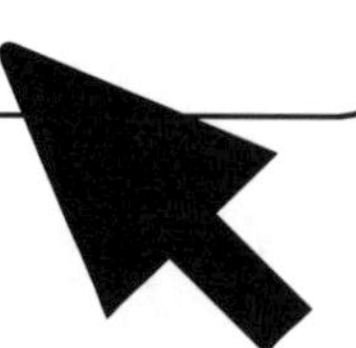

**Thank you for purchasing this product!**

HCPro

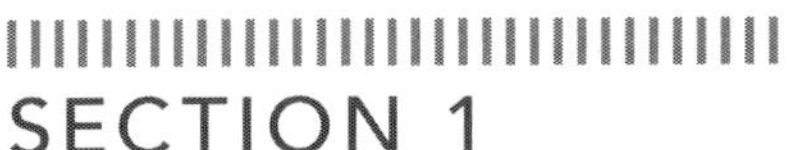

SECTION 1

# Addressing the Preliminaries

Few specific elements contained within the typical set of medical staff bylaws are required by a law, regulation, or accreditation standard. Rather, laws and regulations require medical staffs to address some issues in the bylaws, but how those issues are addressed is up to each medical staff. In fact, the contents of medical staff bylaws are largely discretionary and within the control of the medical staff. Medical staffs often defer to previously published model bylaws that may not reflect contemporary needs and concepts.

For example, many medical staff bylaws include the organization's name, a table of contents, definitions, and a preamble/statement of purpose. Consider whether your medical staff should take a traditional or alternative approach to these bylaws elements.

## Organization Name

Because conventional methods argue that there should always be an article in the bylaws that states the organization's name, chances are that your bylaws contain such language. However, there is no requirement that states that your bylaws must include this article. Therefore, your medical staff could opt to place the name of the organization only on the cover sheet of the bylaws. Using a two-sentence article to restate the organization's name is a waste of time and space and adds to the complexity of the document. Do away with it and you are on your way to more streamlined bylaws.

## Table of Contents

The traditional approach to bylaws construction places the table of contents at the beginning of the document and enables all parties to quickly locate relevant articles, sections, and provisions. In addition to listing the major headings, some medical staff bylaws' table of contents lists each minor subheading within the document. The result is a lengthy table of contents. Although such a detailed table of contents allows users to identify all sections of the bylaws and their corresponding page numbers, it also creates the impression that the bylaws are a dense and bureaucratic document.

Further, the clerical task of updating the table of contents can be daunting when revisions and amendments change the page numbering of every section. If you choose to follow traditional methods and create a table of contents, consider referencing only the major headings within the bylaws, such as the following:

- Appointment to the medical staff
- Membership responsibilities
- Membership rights
- Medical staff categories
- Medical staff officers
- Conflict resolution
- Method of bylaws adoption
- Investigations and corrective action
- Fair hearings

  

- Credentialing processes
- Organizational structure
- Meetings, quorum, and attendance

If your medical staff seeks to create more user-friendly bylaws, you might consider placing the table of contents at the end of the document rather than the beginning. This change will help ensure that physicians who have an interest in reading the bylaws are not put off by first having to wade through a lengthy contents section.

Another option to consider is giving new applicants a summary of the medical staff bylaws. This could be written in a narrative style with a less formal tone that increases the likelihood that physicians will read it. It should serve as the physicians' introduction to the medical staff structure and processes. New physicians should also be directed to a complete set of medical staff bylaws available on the hospital's website, CD, or through the medical staff services department. The medical staff can maintain additional copies of current bylaws in the physician lounge/medical staff library.

## Definitions

Most medical staff bylaws contain a section labeled "definitions." This section of the bylaws can be pared down to save physicians time and create a more user-friendly document. In reality, few physicians are interested in exploring the detailed definition of the word "appointee," or the phrase "special notice."

However, bylaws traditionally include a detailed section at the beginning of the document that precisely defines many of the terms used within. Bylaws committees should, at minimum, refrain from creating a long and immaterial list of definitions. Any word used in the bylaws document that has a commonly accepted definition does not need to be further defined in the bylaws (e.g., corrective action, peer review, governing body, CEO). In addition, words that are defined within the bylaws, such as “special notice,” do not need to be redefined in this section. Names of laws or entities, such as the National Practitioner Data Bank, also do not need to be redefined. An exception is the word “investigation.” For more information on why it is important to clearly define this term, see Section 3.

Your organization’s legal counsel may be uncomfortable omitting the definitions section. If a definitions section must be included, consider designing it so that it does not add to the bureaucratic look of the document. Instead of placing it at the beginning of the bylaws, consider including it at the end, along with the table of contents or other nonessential items.

## Preamble and Statement of Purpose

Many bylaws documents begin with a preamble. If the document includes a preamble, the medical staff should customize it to reflect the unique attributes of the hospital, community, and medical staff, as well as the particular purpose for which the medical staff bylaws have been created. This section is largely an adornment that adds little substantive value to the overall document, and the medical staff can eliminate it. Although some may wish to maintain this introduction to set the stage for the contents that follow, it is best to eliminate excess verbiage whenever possible. The preamble is largely a function of tradition, and there is no requirement for its inclusion. Further, it adds no legal protection and usually does not establish any duty or responsibility that is not otherwise documented.

Another common starting point for medical staff bylaws is a statement of the organization’s purpose and basic responsibilities. You should carefully review this section of your bylaws in light of today’s litigious environment and the realities of current medical practice. Avoid promises that the “purpose of the staff is to provide the highest quality patient care” or “to ensure that only competent practitioners are permitted to provide services within the facility.”

  

A medical staff may certainly strive to achieve these goals, but it is not wise to insert such guarantees into bylaws. Too often, a plaintiff's attorney will search for this language to demonstrate that the medical staff failed to carry out its promise to the board. The purpose of the medical staff is not to make guarantees—it is to ensure that patient care is constantly reviewed, evaluated, and improved when necessary.

Look at your current language. If there is language in the statement of purpose that is later reiterated, then the language in the statement of purpose is unnecessary.

## SAMPLE BYLAWS LANGUAGE

### Purpose and authority

#### Purpose

The purpose of this medical staff is to organize the activities of physicians and other clinical practitioners who practice at XYZ Hospital to carry out, in conformity with these bylaws, the functions delegated to the medical staff by the hospital board.

#### Authority

Subject to the authority and approval of the board, the medical staff will exercise such power as is reasonably necessary to discharge its responsibilities under these bylaws and under the corporate bylaws of the hospital.

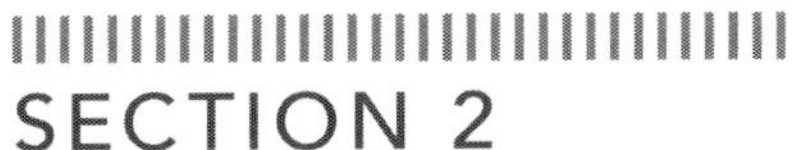

SECTION 2

# Medical Staff Governance

The Joint Commission (TJC) states under MS.01.01.01 that medical staff bylaws must articulate the organization's essential structure and principles of governance.

In this section, we describe various approaches to governance and structure that medical staffs across the United States have experimented with in an effort to increase the value and effectiveness of their organizations. In general, the approaches we outline are meant for a democratically organized medical staff, as this mode of governance predominates in community hospitals across the nation. However, note that many effective medical staffs, especially those at academic medical centers, are not organized democratically and have appointed leadership positions.

There is no one-size-fits-all strategy or single best practice that every medical staff should adopt. In the approaches discussed later in this section, there is no effort to catalog the full range of design options for medical staff governance or the many options for medical staff structure and processes that exist.

When drafting bylaws language, it is always wise to remember the adage "form follows function" and create the most user-friendly and effective approaches.

# Medical Staff Membership

During a hospital stay, patients may encounter—in addition to physicians—advanced practice nurses (APRN), physician assistants (PA), podiatrists, chiropractors, acupuncturists, psychologists, optometrists, and many other practitioners who compose the alphabet soup of clinicians who have permission to work at that institution. Let's start with the basics: Which of these practitioners should be members of the medical staff?

Today, more so than ever, it is important to clearly distinguish between medical staff membership and clinical privileges. The medical staff can recommend that the board grant a physician membership but not privileges. For example, it is common for medical staffs to grant retired, distinguished physicians membership on the medical staff in an honorary category, but not to grant them privileges to directly manage inpatient care. Alternatively, Joint Commission standards require that certain practitioners—such as APRNs and PAs—be granted privileges, even though they are commonly not eligible to become members of the medical staff.

In addition to physicians (MD or DO), it is also common to see medical staff membership granted to podiatrists, dentists, and oral/maxillofacial surgeons. Beyond this grouping, there is wide variation in the types of practitioners who are allowed medical staff membership. For example, some states mandate that certain practitioners, such as psychologists, be eligible for medical staff membership. Thus, it is always best to check your state's requirements before writing a bylaws provision.

More medical staffs are considering whether to include podiatrists, psychologists, PAs, and APRNs on their medical staffs. These practitioners are vital parts of the provider community, and some medical staffs want to recognize this through medical staff membership. However, by granting these practitioners medical staff membership, they receive the same medical staff rights as all other members of the medical staff, including fair hearing and appeal rights.

  

Nonphysician, non-dentist practitioners who are medical staff members receive the full legalistic and bureaucratic fair hearing and appeal process as physicians and dentists. The Health Care Quality Improvement Act of 1986 (HCQIA) requires that medical staffs provide this fair hearing process to physicians and dentists for hospitals to receive immunity protections under the law. If nonphysician and non-dentist practitioners are privileged but not members of the medical staff, the medical staff can devise a simple method of fair hearing and appeal. It is a cultural choice (unless mandated by state law) whether these other practitioners should become medical staff members.

Practitioners on the medical staff are granted the rights and protections of the medical staff bylaws and are permitted to participate in whatever activities their staff category permits. Once you determine which practitioners are eligible for medical staff membership, the bylaws should clearly list the appropriate professional groups that may apply.

## SAMPLE BYLAWS LANGUAGE

### Medical staff membership

Membership on the medical staff of XYZ Hospital is a privilege that shall be extended only to professionally competent physicians, dentists, and [list any others as appropriate] who continuously meet the qualifications, standards, and requirements set forth in these bylaws and the associated policies of the medical staff and hospital.

## Membership Responsibilities

There is no way to enumerate all the responsibilities of medical staff members in the bylaws. However, you can categorize them under some useful headings and put more detail in associated documents if necessary.

Usually, the most common responsibilities found in bylaws require medical staff members to:

- Provide appropriate, timely, and continuous care of patients
- Participate in quality/peer review activities
- Submit to a pertinent health exam when requested as it relates to safely exercising one's privileges
- Abide by the bylaws, rules and regulations, and policies and procedures of the medical staff and the hospital
- Purchase professional liability coverage that is deemed adequate for the organization
- Maintain confidentiality according to the Health Insurance Portability and Accountability Act of 1996 (HIPAA)
- Complete medical records in a legible and timely manner
- Participate in emergency department (ED) call coverage consistent with clinical privileges

Two items to note: The Centers for Medicare & Medicaid Services (CMS) requires medical staff bylaws address who can perform the history and physical examination and in what time frame the history and physical exam must be completed.

  

## SAMPLE BYLAWS LANGUAGE

### Completion of history and physical examinations

A medical history and physical examination must be completed no more than 30 days before or 24 hours after admission or registration, but prior to surgery, an interventional diagnostic procedure, or a procedure requiring anesthesia services. The medical history and physical examination must be completed and documented by a physician, an oral/maxillofacial surgeon, or other qualified licensed individual in accordance with state law and hospital policy.

An updated examination of the patient, including any changes in the patient's condition, must be completed and documented within 24 hours after admission or registration, but prior to surgery, an interventional diagnostic procedure, or a procedure requiring anesthesia services, when the medical history and physical examination is completed within 30 days before admission or registration. The updated examination of the patient, including any changes in the patient's condition, must be completed and documented by a physician, an oral/maxillofacial surgeon, or other qualified licensed individual in accordance with state law and hospital policy.

The other item that needs to be addressed is ED call coverage. When responsibilities like ED coverage are assigned to specific medical staff categories, some physicians may intentionally switch categories to avoid the burden of this responsibility. As a result, medical staff leaders may find that their bylaws hinder their ability to effectively carry out the organization's responsibilities. Therefore, this responsibility is best addressed using general language. General language makes ED call everyone's responsibility—and the medical executive committee (MEC) can assign that responsibility after it carefully studies the variables related to this issue at the hospital. The MEC has the ability to address the issue free from the arbitrary shackles of category assigments.

SAMPLE BYLAWS LANGUAGE

**Emergency department call**

Staff members, consistent with their granted clinical privileges, must participate in the on-call coverage of the emergency department or in other hospital coverage programs as determined by the MEC and the board, after receiving input from the appropriate clinical specialty.

## Membership Rights

Just as medical staff members have responsibilities, they also have rights. Member rights tend to be scattered throughout the bylaws document. They range from the rights of individuals to receive a fair hearing and appeal to the right of the organized medical staff to question rules or policies promulgated by the MEC.

The rights of members vary from medical staff to medical staff, but they tend to include the following:

- Individual rights
  - The right to meet with the MEC on matters relevant to the responsibilities of the MEC that may affect patient care or safety if the medical staff is unable to resolve the issue with the department chair
  - The right to fair hearing and appeal (addressed further in Section 3)

  

- Group rights (with appropriate number of signatures on petition)
  - The right to initiate a recall after an election of officers
  - The right to initiate a recall after an election of department chairs
  - The right to initiate a call for a general staff meeting
  - The right to initiate a call for a department meeting
  - The right to challenge any rule or policy adopted by the MEC

## Medical Staff Categories

Most medical staff bylaws contain a substantial provision concerning the categories into which the staff will be divided. Many medical staffs have created an unnecessarily complex array of categories. Why? The number of categories expanded in the 1970s and 1980s as staffs tried to accommodate various individual physician situations. Medical staffs create categories in an attempt to answer questions such as these:

- In what category do we put the hand surgeon who practices at the hospital a couple of times a year?
- In what category do we put the specialist who infrequently performs consults?
- In what category do we put the community-based no-volume or low-volume provider who may no longer be able to demonstrate current clinical competence to maintain inpatient privileges?
- Which practitioners (in which categories) should be required to take ED call?

  

Some medical staffs function effectively with only two categories, whereas others are carrying the bureaucratic weight of more than 10.

CMS' *Conditions of Participation* (*CoP*) require hospitals to provide a statement of the duties and privileges of each medical staff category. In addition to meeting CMS' *CoPs*, most medical staffs create categories for two reasons. The first and most important is to determine the citizenship status of various members of the medical staff. A member category indicates whether a practitioner can vote in general medical staff elections or on bylaws amendments, serve as an officer of the organization, sit and vote on committees, and so forth. The other reason is to assign certain responsibilities—such as ED or clinic coverage—to practitioners based on their category. Again, ED coverage is a general responsibility of all medical staff members based on clinical privileges and should not be the subject of category determination.

## *Inclusive versus exclusive medical staffs*

If categories are reserved for articulating citizenship duties, how many categories are necessary? If we use the Einstein quote "All things should be made as simple as possible but not more so," then most staffs could get by with just two or three categories. The active category is typically reserved for staff members who are entitled to hold elected officer positions/vote at general medical staff, department, and committee meetings and on bylaws amendments. Traditionally, the eligibility criteria for active staff membership were based on the number of patient contacts a physician had at the hospital. If a medical staff feels that only physicians who care for a significant number of patients at the hospital should have a say in how the medical staff is run, it is being somewhat exclusive.

Some medical staffs look at the evolving medical landscape and see family practice and internal medicine physicians who are no longer busy in the hospital, but who refer hundreds of patients to the hospital and its staff physicians. The medical staffs may view these physicians as an integral part of the institution and want them to stay involved in medical staff affairs if they so desire. These medical staffs are considered inclusive.

  

Deciding whether your medical staff wants to be inclusive or exclusive will help you set the requirements for the active category. Usually two elements come into play—a physician's activity (or number of contacts) and his or her engagement in medical staff affairs if he or she does not have a significant number of patient contacts.

Exclusivists argue that only someone who practices within the hospital should be allowed to vote and affect the activities of other providers. Otherwise, there would be members voting on issues that don't affect them because they do not have significant activity in the hospital. This is a valid argument.

Inclusivists argue that everyone who is cognizant of the activities in the hospital, either through direct patient care or through attendance at meetings, should be allowed to vote. They also argue that primary care physicians who send their patients to hospitalists still care about the quality of care that their patients receive at the hospital. Again, this is a valid argument.

Rarely do medical staffs not allow low- and no-volume physicians (primarily outpatient physicians who refer their patients to hospitalists) to be members—medical staffs want these practitioners to be engaged in hospital activities and want them to continue to refer patients to the hospital. The contentious issue is whether low- and no-volume physicians should have a vote. As noted earlier, each side has valid arguments. All parties should openly discuss their preferences with each other and make a cultural decision.

A middle ground could be called the "earn a vote" position. This position allows members who have knowledge of the workings of the medical staff to have a vote; they are thought to have the knowledge to make intelligent decisions. They can demonstrate this knowledge either through sufficient clinical activity at the organization or through attendance/participation at a predefined number of medical staff meetings.

Another issue that comes into play is practitioners' tenure on the medical staff. Some medical staffs feel that members should be on the medical staff for a minimum amount of time before they are afforded the opportunity to vote and hold office. For example, these medical staffs may require a one- to two-year tenure on the medical staff before the member is eligible for the active category and receives the option to vote. Other staffs give members voting rights immediately, not wishing to disenfranchise someone who has made a commitment to work at the hospital.

## *Common medical staff categories*

**Active category:** This category typically includes physicians who have been on the medical staff for a reasonable time period and who are active and interested in the institution's clinical affairs, as noted by clinical activity, engagement in medical staff affairs (i.e., meeting attendance), or other parameters. Establishing clear criteria for inclusion in this category minimizes the complexity and confusion that occasionally surrounds the issue.

Physicians in this category are allowed to do the following:

- Members can attend medical staff or department meetings of which they are a member, as well as any medical staff or hospital education programs

- Members vote on all matters presented by the medical staff, department, or committee(s) to which the members are assigned

- Members [can/cannot] hold office and sit on or be the chair of any committee in accordance with any qualifying criteria set forth elsewhere in the medical staff bylaws or medical staff policies

The responsibilities of this category are usually the general membership responsibilities noted earlier in this section.

  

**Associate category:** Associate staff members are typically interested in remaining members of the medical staff but do not meet the requirements for the active category. Often, physicians who are new to the medical staff are made associate members. In addition, longtime medical staff members who are not active (and are non-voting members) or who are not interested in participating in the organization's affairs can be placed in this category.

The prerogatives of this category could include the following:

- Members can attend medical staff or department meetings of which they are a member, as well as any medical staff or hospital education programs
- Members cannot vote on matters before the entire medical staff or be an officer of the medical staff
- Members [can/cannot] serve on medical staff committees other than the MEC and may vote on matters that come before such committees

The responsibilities of this category are usually the general membership responsibilities noted earlier in this section.

**Affiliate (community-based) category:** The affiliate category is usually reserved for members who maintain a clinical practice in the hospital service area and wish to follow their patients when they are admitted to the hospital.

The prerogatives of this category could include the following:

- Members can order noninvasive outpatient diagnostic tests and services; visit patients in the hospital; review medical records; and attend medical staff or department meetings, continuing medical education (CME) functions, and social events
- Members cannot be eligible for clinical privileges and cannot manage patient care in the hospital
- Members [can/cannot] vote on medical staff affairs or hold office depending on the decision the medical staff has made regarding the inclusiveness or exclusiveness of the medical staff

Because the members of this category do not hold any clinical privileges, their responsibilities are restricted other than to fulfill or comply with any applicable medical staff or hospital policies and procedures.

**Honorary category:** Physicians who the staff and board wish to honor for past service are frequently appointed to the honorary medical staff.

The prerogatives of this category could include the following:

- Members may attend medical staff or department meetings, as well as CME activities
- Members may be appointed to committees, but they shall not hold clinical privileges, hold office, or be eligible to vote

Because the members of this category do not hold any clinical privileges, their responsibilities are restricted other than to fulfill or comply with any applicable medical staff or hospital policies and procedures.

## Medical Staff Officers

The officers of the staff should govern and effectuate the administrative functions of the medical staff. As the relationships between clinicians and hospitals become increasingly complex and contentious, it is more important than ever that qualified officers lead the medical staff.

Fifty years ago, the office of the medical staff president or chief of staff was an honorary position that required little work. There weren't many committees to serve on or specific regulatory requirements or standards to meet. There was no such thing as "managed care," "pay for performance," or even Medicare and Medicaid. Physicians practiced at the hospital regularly and did not have to contend with the complex legal and medical malpractice issues they face today.

  

In addition, physicians were respected by their patients and society in general and enjoyed allegiances that were aligned more fully with those of the hospital. There were no real selection criteria to become an officer, short of being on the active staff and breathing. Hospitals did little in the way of succession planning and often selected leaders using the "next in the barrel" philosophy. People were nominated for officer positions from the floor, regardless of whether they had the desire, experience, or time to do the job.

In today's complex healthcare environment, it is becoming increasingly difficult to find physicians who want to get involved in medical staff leadership positions. However, it is more important than ever to recruit, educate, train, and retain strong medical staff leaders. In a section dealing with medical staff officers, the bylaws must address the following factors:

- Number of officers on the medical staff
- Description of each officer's role
- Duration of term in office
- Required qualifications or selection criteria, if applicable
- Nomination and election processes
- Conditions for recall or removal of officers

Let's examine each of these issues in more detail.

## *Number of officers on the medical staff*

All medical staffs have either a president or chief of staff—same position, different names. For simplicity, this book will refer to this officer as the president of the medical staff.

  

Most medical staffs also have *either* a vice president or a president-elect. What is the difference? If the president can no longer continue to serve in the position, a vice president takes over until the current term expires. In addition, the vice president assists the president on request. A president-elect not only takes over if the president can no longer continue in the job, but he or she also becomes the next president at the end of the current term. Having a president-elect instead of a vice-president ensures continuity in the cohort of officers and allows an experienced individual to step into this important medical staff role.

However, having a president-elect has the potential downside of locking someone into position who may not be the ideal candidate for president. For example, this person may have been controversial as the president-elect; had a consuming life event, such as a divorce or illness; experienced a change in practice circumstances, leaving little time for medical staff responsibilities; or became an employee of a competing health center. Under such circumstances, automatic ascendancy into the role of president may be less than desirable.

Some medical staffs have a secretary/treasurer position and use this role as an opportunity to groom future leaders. Other staffs have eliminated this position altogether because, in today's environment, the tasks of taking minutes and collecting money typically fall to MSPs. Still others have revised the role to give it a more contemporary purpose. For example, they may rename the role from treasurer or secretary to "medical staff communications officer" to ensure that effective communication occurs among all medical staff members.

Most medical staffs wish to benefit from the education, training, and experience of immediate past presidents. Thus, they consider these individuals as officers.

I generally see at least two officers on most medical staffs (the president and vice president or president-elect). However, I have seen up to four officers (the president, vice president or president-elect, secretary/treasurer, and immediate past president).

  

## *Description of each officer's role*

Typically, only a brief description of each officer's role is included in the bylaws because some of these descriptions, especially the medical staff president's, can be quite lengthy. Every medical staff should provide elsewhere clear job descriptions that enumerate each officer's duties and performance expectations. Complete job descriptions can be exhibits to the bylaws or be included in policy manuals or in other associated medical staff documents.

In short, the president is the primary elected officer of the medical staff, serving as the medical staff's advocate and representative to the board and hospital administration. The president usually serves as the chair of the MEC and an ex officio member of all other medical staff committees, participating (when invited) on board or hospital committees. The president is responsible for enforcing the medical staff bylaws; regularly evaluates the effectiveness of the hospital's credentialing and privileging processes; and reports results to the board, the MEC, and administration. It is customary for the president to appoint committee chairs and members.

In the absence of the president, the vice president or president-elect assumes all the duties of the president. This person is a member of the MEC. Some staffs require the vice president or president-elect to chair either the medical staff quality/peer review committee or the credentials committee. This practice enhances his or her leadership training and also forces these vital committees to have rotational leadership every two years. As a leading practice, hospitals may require the vice president or president-elect to at least be a member of one or both of these committees at some point during his or her term, but it does not allow him or her to serve as chair. This allows the committee to be chaired with continuity by an individual who has valuable expertise and experience in the affairs of that committee while allowing the vice president or president-elect to gain needed experience.

The secretary/treasurer (if the office exists) is also a member of the MEC and may sit on additional medical staff committees. As noted, members of the medical staff have a harder time communicating today because they come to the hospital for meetings far less than in the past years. Thus, the secretary/treasurer's responsibility to maintain medical staff communications is crucial.

The immediate past president is frequently a member of the MEC and may serve as the chair of the nominating committee to help identify future officers and medical staff leaders. In many cases, the immediate past president also serves in a mentoring role for current medical staff leaders. Many staffs feel that the expertise of the immediate past president makes him or her well suited to be a member or chair of the credentials committee. As a best practice, strive for continuity in the credentials chair position—do not mandate that the past president chair this important committee.

### *Duration of term in office*

The bylaws must describe the term of office for each position. Many medical staffs believe that a one-year term of office is too short. As president, it may take six months or longer to understand how things really work, let alone get anything accomplished. A three- or four-year term seems to be too long of a commitment for most physicians. As a result, many staffs settle on a two-year term of office.

A common question among medical staffs is whether any officer (or the president) should be allowed to run for more than one term in office. Proponents say that an officer who is doing a good job, wants to continue, and has the support of the medical staff should be allowed to run for a second or third term. They ask, why let a bylaws requirement force a medical staff to lose the leadership of a skilled officer? (Of course, this might not be an option if you have a president-elect.) Other staffs believe that strict term limits enable fresh ideas to be heard, prevent the creation of leadership cliques, and inject more medical staff members into leadership roles. This is a cultural decision that each medical staff must make.

The bylaws must describe the following:

- The qualifications for officer positions
- How officers are elected
- How vacancies in office will be handled
- A mechanism and conditions under which the medical staff can remove an officer

  

## *Qualifications or selection criteria*

Hospitals with well-defined leadership selection criteria that establish a physician's eligibility to run for office are more likely to elect well-qualified, committed, and knowledgeable medical staff officers. It is hard to hit the target unless you aim for it. Medical staffs have been expanding the list of job eligibility requirements to include some or all of the following criteria:

- The physician must be an active staff member in good standing for a certain number of years. In this context, a physician in "good standing" has a record free of adverse recommendations concerning medical staff appointments/privileges, license/Drug Enforcement Agency sanctions, and professional conduct or quality issues.

- The physician has several years' experience in a medical staff leadership position or equivalent (e.g., the physician has served as a department or committee chair or as a member of the executive committee).

- The physician has received medical staff leadership training or demonstrates a willingness to attend such training three to five days per year.

- The physician agrees not to be a medical staff or board leader at any other competing facility during his or her term in office.

- The physician fully discloses all conflicts of interest or interest in competing healthcare entities.

- The physician recognizes and agrees to the commitment of time needed to perform the duties associated with the role and assumes responsibility for participating in continuing leadership education.

- The physician demonstrates the ability to work positively and communicate well with colleagues, hospital administration, and the board.

  

CMS requires that the president of the medical staff be a physician, dentist, or podiatrist. Therefore, if you allow other practitioners to be members of the medical staff, you will need to add this specific qualification to the position of president of the medical staff (and to the president-elect of the medical staff due to the automatic succession to the office of the president).

### *Nomination and election process*

To avoid nominating someone from the floor at the last minute who does not have the experience, desire, or time to hold an officer's position, most staffs have a nominating committee composed of MEC members/at-large medical staff members. Many staffs have the immediate past president chair the committee, or they construct the committee entirely of former officers. The committee meets before the anticipated election and, using preestablished selection criteria, nominates at least one candidate for each available position.

If a hospital chooses to create a nominating committee, the bylaws should articulate the process for choosing nominees and disseminating information about the running slate. For example, the bylaws might require the nominating committee to distribute the present ballot of candidates to the entire medical staff (by posting it in the physicians' lounges, via direct mail, etc.) at least 30 days prior to the election. The bylaws might allow additional nominations on the ballot if a certain percentage of the active medical staff signs a petition. Bylaws could also require the active medical staff to submit such a petition to the nominating committee at least 14 days prior to the election, allowing time for the nominating committee to verify that the candidate meets the qualifications required to run for office. Although not a regulatory requirement, this is a leading practice.

This approach enables a medical staff member to nominate any candidate but creates a screening process to ensure that the candidate meets the predetermined selection criteria that the medical staff has agreed on. In general, medical staffs should avoid the practice of nominating officers from the floor. Because the task of finding, educating, training, and retaining strong medical staff leaders is becoming increasingly important, consider establishing an ongoing leadership and succession planning committee. This committee develops selection criteria, outlines a leadership training process, and creates a pool of future leaders. The details of this committee are discussed further in Section 6.

Two common approaches to electing officers exist: a vote by those present at a meeting or some type of mail ballot.

Many medical staffs like the feel of town hall meetings, where direct discussion can occur. Typically, elections are held at an annual medical staff meeting. Because medical staffs are required to meet at least once a year, the turnout is likely to be higher for elections held during these annual meetings.

If your medical staff conducts an election during a meeting, you must decide whether only those present at the meeting can vote or whether the medical staff will accept absentee or proxy votes. If only two candidates are running, the candidate who receives the most votes wins. If more than two candidates are running, your medical staff must decide whether the candidate with the most votes wins or whether a candidate is required to obtain a majority vote (50% plus one) to be elected. If your medical staff decides that the candidate must receive a majority vote, you must create a plan for a run-off election. Usually, run-off elections involve dropping the candidate with the lowest vote total and voting again until one candidate obtains a majority vote.

Another approach is to provide a mail-in ballot to all eligible members of the medical staff and require them to return the ballots by a certain date (usually five to 30 days prior to the end of the term). This eliminates any absentee or proxy vote concerns. Some technology-savvy medical staffs allow staff members to vote using various electronic means (e.g., by email, on a website, by fax, or even by telephone). Regardless of the voting method you choose, your medical staff still must determine whether a candidate needs a majority vote to be elected. If so, a run-off election process must be described in the bylaws.

Many medical staffs are now electing MEC at-large members (to be discussed further in this section) using many of the same selection criteria and election processes that apply to the officers. These MEC at-large members are another way to allow the general medical staff to elect individuals who are not officers to represent the entire medical staff instead of separate department constituencies.

### *Conditions for recall or removal of officers*

The medical staff bylaws must describe a process for removing medical staff officers from

SAMPLE BYLAWS LANGUAGE

## Medical staff officers

Officers of the medical staff (and MEC at-large members)

- President of the medical staff
- Vice president of the medical staff
- Secretary/treasurer/communications officer
- Immediate past president

### Qualifications of officers (and MEC at-large members)

Officers and MEC at-large members must be members of the active category in good standing for [X] years and be actively involved in patient care in the hospital. They must have previously served in a significant leadership position on a medical staff

SAMPLE BYLAWS LANGUAGE

## Medical staff officers (cont.)

(e.g., department chair, committee chair), indicate a willingness and ability to serve, have no pending adverse recommendations concerning medical staff appointment or clinical privileges, have participated in medical staff leadership training and/or be willing to participate in such training during their term of office, have demonstrated an ability to work well with others, be in compliance with the professional conduct policies of the hospital, and have excellent administrative and communication skills. The medical staff leadership and succession planning committee will have discretion to determine if a staff member wishing to run for office meets the qualifying criteria.

Officers and MEC at-large members may not simultaneously hold a leadership position on another hospital's medical staff or in a facility that directly competes with the hospital. Noncompliance with this requirement will result in the officer being automatically removed from office unless the board determines that allowing the officer to maintain the position is in the best interest of the hospital. The board shall have discretion to determine what constitutes a "leadership position" at another hospital.

***Election of officers and MEC at-large members***

The leadership and succession planning committee shall offer at least one nominee for each available position. Nominations must be announced and the names of the nominees distributed to all members of the active medical staff at least 30 days prior to the election.

A petition signed by at least [X%] of the members of the active staff may add nominations to the ballot. The medical staff must submit such a petition to the medical staff president at least 14 days prior to the election for the nominee(s) to be placed on the ballot. The leadership and succession committee must determine if candidates meet

SAMPLE BYLAWS LANGUAGE

## Medical staff officers (cont.)

the qualifications in the section of the bylaws that address qualifications of offers and MEC at-large members before they can be placed on the ballot.

New officers and MEC at-large members shall be elected at least one month prior to the expiration of the term of the current officers. Only members of the active category shall be eligible to vote. The MSP will determine the mechanisms by which votes may be cast, subject to the approval of the MEC. The mechanisms that may be considered include written mail ballots and electronic voting via computer, fax, or other technology for transmitting the members' voting choices. No proxy voting will be permissible. The nominee with the greatest number/majority of votes will be elected. In the event of a vote without a clear winner, the MSP will make arrangements for repeat votes until one candidate receives the required number of votes.

### *Term of office*

All officers and MEC at-large members serve a term of two years. They shall take office in the month of [X]. An individual [may/may not] be re-elected for two successive terms.

### *Vacancies of office*

The MEC shall fill vacancies of office during the medical staff year, which may vary from the calendar year (e.g., Nov. 1–Oct. 31), except the office of the medical staff president. If there is a vacancy in the office of the medical staff president, the vice president shall serve the remainder of the term.

  

SAMPLE BYLAWS LANGUAGE

## Medical staff officers (cont.)

### Duties of officers (and MEC at-large members):

**President:** The president shall represent the interests of the medical staff to the MEC and the board. The president will fulfill the duties specified in Section [X] of these bylaws (the organization and functions manual).

**Vice president:** In the absence of the president, the vice president shall assume all the duties and have the authority of the president. The vice president shall perform additional duties to assist the president as requested.

**Secretary/treasurer/communications officer:** This officer collaborates with the hospital's medical staff services department, ensures maintenance of minutes, attends to correspondence, acts as medical staff treasurer, and coordinates communication within the medical staff. This person shall perform additional duties to assist the president as requested.

**Immediate past president:** This officer will serve as a consultant to the president and vice president and provide feedback to the officers regarding their performance of assigned duties on an annual basis. This person shall perform additional duties to assist the president as requested.

**MEC at-large members:** These members will advise and support the medical staff officers and are responsible for representing the needs/interests of the entire medical staff, not simply representing the preferences of their own clinical specialty.

office, should the need arise. Having such a method in place not only makes sense, but it is also required by accreditation agencies, especially if the officer has failed to comply with the requirements of the position. Consider instituting automatic removal criteria for events such as the following:

- Suspension of clinical privileges lasting more than 30 days

- Failure to comply with medical staff bylaws or hospital policies and procedures
- Conduct or statements that are damaging to the hospital and the medical staff
- A felony conviction

In circumstances other than those necessitating automatic removal of an officer, the MEC or general medical staff may want to remove an officer. Many staffs rely on a two-thirds affirmative vote by the MEC to remove a member. In addition, consider instituting a process whereby a petition signed by a certain percentage (e.g., 20%) of the active medical staff and an affirmative two-thirds vote by the entire staff would result in the removal of an officer from the medical staff. Department chairs could be removed via a similar process, except the vote would be limited to members of their respective departments.

## SAMPLE BYLAWS LANGUAGE

### Removal from office

The medical staff may remove any officer or MEC at-large member if at least [X%] of the active staff members sign a petition advocating such action. The petition must be followed by an affirmative two-thirds vote of those active staff members casting ballot votes. Members of the MEC will automatically be removed if they fail to meet the responsibilities assigned to them within these bylaws or fail to comply with policies and procedures of the medical staff. Members can also be removed for conduct or statements that damage the hospital, its goals, or programs or for an automatic or precautionary suspension of clinical privileges that lasts more than 30 days. After consulting with the joint conference committee, the board will determine if members have failed in their duties.

*Author's note: Most bylaws that I review contain a conflict resolution mechanism for when issues need to be addressed between the MEC and the board. This conflict resolution mechanism is usually a committee comprised of an equal number of individuals from both bodies, usually called the Joint Conference Committee.*

  

## The Medical Executive Committee

CMS does not require any medical staff committees, even an MEC. In fact, Det Norske Veritas (DNV), the Healthcare Facilities Accreditation Program of the American Osteopathic Association (HFAP), and the Center for Improvement in Healthcare Quality (CIHQ), which closely follow CMS' *CoPs*, do not require an MEC but do state that if one exists, the majority of its members must be physicians or dentists. Contrary to these other accrediting agencies, TJC requires medical staffs to have MECs. It's standard MS.01.01.01 states that medical staff bylaws must include the MEC's function, size, and composition. The bylaws should also describe the authority delegated to the MEC by the organized medical staff to act on its behalf.

The composition of the MEC is established in the medical staff bylaws and varies widely from hospital to hospital. Some have small, efficient MECs comprising four or five members, whereas others have 25 or more members. Many are largely composed of the chairs of departments, whereas others are mostly made up of members elected at large.

Although department chairs comprise the MEC at most hospitals, it is worth emphasizing that no regulatory body requires such a model. Many medical staffs believe that allowing department chairs representation on the MEC is fundamentally unfair because doing so allots the same MEC vote to a four-person department as a 70-person department. Others are rethinking the traditional link between department chairs and the MEC because of the difficulty of finding qualified leaders in every department.

Many practitioners are elected as department chairs because they failed to attend the department meeting at which elections were held. When this occurs, the MEC will likely have members who are not interested in broad medical staff affairs or not particularly skillful in dealing with them.

  

Another criticism of electing department chairs to the MEC is that doing so promotes a "silo" mentality in which members see themselves as defenders of their specialty's interests rather than contributors to the effectiveness of the entire medical staff. In effect, they are union reps rather than statespersons.

Such criticisms beg the question, then, of how a medical staff should construct the MEC. Medical staffs grapple with the following questions about the MEC:

- Which individuals should be on the MEC?
- How large should the committee be?
- Should members be elected or appointed?
- What ex officio members do we need on the committee?
- How are MEC members removed?
- What functions will be required of the MEC, and what duties does TJC require?

Let's look at these questions in more detail.

### *Which individuals should be on the MEC?*

An effective medical staff must do three things well:

- Govern itself
- Make recommendations regarding the credentialing and privileging of practitioners
- Monitor the quality of care provided by practitioners

Keeping these three tasks in mind can help you decide who should serve on the MEC. Most medical staffs elect officers, and these officers are a logical first choice when considering

  

MEC membership. Many medical staffs believe that because credentialing and quality monitoring are important tasks—and much of the MEC's business revolves around these two functions—it is prudent to have the chairs of the credentials committee and the medical staff quality/peer review committee sit on the MEC as well. These individuals might be present with a vote or may just be regular guests at MEC meetings.

## *How large should the committee be?*

Who else should serve on the MEC? This question may depend on how big the medical staff wants the MEC to be. The most effective size for a decision-making body is five to seven people—big enough to ensure various opinions and robust discussion, but not big enough to thwart constructive, give-and-take conversation.

Some medical staffs may think that five to seven members may be too small, but most believe an MEC larger than 15 members is too unruly and unproductive. Thus, many medical staffs maintain an MEC of eight to 12 members. By setting an approximate target number, which would include medical staff officers and possibly the credentials chair and medical staff quality/peer review committee chair, you can better decide how to assemble the other members of the MEC.

For example, the other members could be elected at large by the entire medical staff. To promote broad representation, medical staffs may require that MEC members are drawn at large from various disciplines (e.g., at least one from a medical specialty and at least one from a surgical specialty). Physicians at these institutions often feel this is a more democratic structure than the more traditional MEC, which consists primarily of department chairs.

## *Should members be elected or appointed?*

If a reasonably modest number of clinical departments exist on a medical staff, it may be appropriate for the medical staff to automatically appoint all department chairs to the MEC. If a large number of departments exist, appointing all of the chairs may create an unwieldy MEC, so an election of MEC members may be more appropriate. At some hospitals, department chairs are appointed, yet at other hospitals, the members of the department elect them. This may be a factor in determining which chairs should sit on the MEC.

### *What ex officio members do we need on the committee?*

The Joint Commission's standard MS.02.01.01 EP 2 states that the MEC must have the hospital's CEO or a designee present in an ex officio capacity, with or without voting rights. DNV requires that if the medical staff has an MEC, the CEO and the chief nurse executive be present in an ex officio capacity, with or without voting rights.

If a hospital employs a vice president of medical affairs (VPMA) or a chief medical officer, it is customary for this individual to sit on the MEC with or without voting rights. Some medical staff bylaws allow the VPMA to serve as the chair of the MEC, recognizing that he or she is usually an experienced physician executive with good meeting management skills.

Many medical staffs also require the chief operating officer, the chief nursing officer, and an MSP to serve as regular ex officio participants without voting rights. This ensures that hospital personnel who can respond to members' questions and concerns are present at MEC meetings.

Finally, TJC requires that the majority of voting MEC members are fully licensed physicians who actively practice at the hospital. HFAP and DNV require that physicians and dentists comprise the majority of the voting members of the MEC, if one is present. CIHQ requires that a majority of the voting members of the MEC, if present, is composed of physicians.

### *How are MEC members removed?*

The medical staff should have a process in place to remove MEC members. Typically, the bylaws contain language addressing the removal of officers and department chairs if the medical staff is departmentalized. However, there must also be a process for removing other elected or appointed members. One method involves the MEC removing the member by a two-thirds vote if the MEC establishes that the member is not fulfilling committee responsibilities. Another method allows elected representatives of the MEC to be removed by a two-thirds supermajority of the same body that elected them originally. Appointees, such as committee chairs or appointed department chairs, could be removed by the same body that originally appointed them.

### *What functions will be required of the MEC, and what duties do the regulatory agencies require?*

Traditionally, the MEC has been the decision-making body of the medical staff—it is the last to rule on matters before they are brought to the board for approval. As a result, the medical staff bylaws should clearly articulate the responsibilities of this committee.

Some of these duties and functions are spelled out in Joint Commission requirements (see standard MS.02.01.01), and they are reflected in the sample bylaws language provided in this book.

SAMPLE BYLAWS LANGUAGE

#### Medical executive committee

**Composition:** The MEC shall be a standing committee consisting of the following voting members: the officers of the medical staff, the chairs of the credentials and quality/peer review committees, the chairs of certain departments, and [X] active medical staff members elected at large. The chair will be the president of the medical staff.

**Removal from MEC:** Officers or department chairs who are removed from their positions in accordance with Section [X] will automatically lose their membership on the MEC. When the chair of either the credentials or quality/peer review committees or a department chair resigns or is removed from these positions, the chair's replacement will serve on the MEC. Other members of the MEC may be removed by a two-thirds affirmative vote of MEC members. When a member of the MEC who was elected at large resigns or is removed, the MEC will arrange for an at-large election for a replacement to serve out the remainder of the vacated term. Such an election will follow procedures established by the MEC and must take place within 60 days of the removal of an MEC member.

## SAMPLE BYLAWS LANGUAGE

### Medical executive committee (cont.)

**Duties:** The duties of the MEC, as delegated by the medical staff, shall be to:

- Serve as the final decision-making body of the medical staff in accordance with the medical staff bylaws and provide oversight for all medical staff functions
- Coordinate the implementation of policies adopted by the board
- Submit recommendations to the board concerning all matters relating to appointment, reappointment, staff category, department assignments, clinical privileges, and corrective action
- Report to the board and to the staff the overall quality and efficiency of professional patient care services provided by individuals with clinical privileges and coordinate the participation of the medical staff in organizational performance improvement activities
- Take reasonable steps to encourage professionally ethical conduct and competent clinical performance on the part of staff members, including collegial and educational efforts and investigations when warranted
- Make recommendations to the board on medical, administrative, and hospital management matters
- Update the medical staff on issues concerning the licensure and accreditation status of the hospital
- Participate in identifying community health needs and setting hospital goals and implementing programs to meet those needs
- Review and act on reports from medical staff committees, departments, and other assigned activity groups
- Formulate and recommend medical staff rules and policies and procedures to the board
- Request evaluations of practitioners privileged through the medical staff process when there is doubt about an applicant or member's ability to perform privileges he or she has requested or currently holds
- Make recommendations concerning the structure of the medical staff, the mechanism by which medical staff membership or privileges may be terminated,

  

SAMPLE BYLAWS LANGUAGE

### Medical executive committee (cont.)

and the mechanisms for fair hearing procedures

- Consult with administration on the quality, timeliness, and appropriateness of contracts for patient care services provided to the hospital by entities outside the hospital
- Oversee the portion of the corporate compliance plan that pertains to the medical staff
- Hold medical staff leaders, committees, and departments accountable for fulfilling their duties and responsibilities
- Make recommendations to the medical staff for changes or amendments to the medical staff bylaws
- Act on behalf of the medical staff between meetings of the medical staff

## Medical Staff Structure: Should the Medical Staff Be Departmentalized?

CMS's *CoPs* state that medical staff bylaws must "describe the organization of the medical staff" (42 *CFR* § 482.22(c)). Likewise, TJC's accreditation standards require that medical staff bylaws include a "definition of the medical staff structure" (see MS.01.01.01 EP 6). So, what should a medical staff consider as it develops this section of its bylaws?

Medical staffs have historically organized themselves around clinical departments. This was initially a relatively simple structure composed of a few key departments representing major specialties, including medicine, surgery, OB-GYN, and—occasionally—pediatrics.

With the explosion of subspecialty medicine after World War II, physicians began to focus on their narrow areas of practice. During the same period, TJC became an increasingly important regulatory organization, issuing standards that focused department activities much more intensely on peer review and credentialing functions. Specialists found that medical staff department meetings involving multiple specialties were less focused on their particular concerns. As a result, they insisted that medical staffs grant them the autonomy to regulate their own affairs, and large departments of medicine and surgery began to develop clinical sections that were subspecialty in nature.

The development of specialties also spurred turf disputes, and physicians formed various opinions about the best way to prioritize and organize hospital services, equipment, and staffing. Soon, clinical sections were demanding representation on the MEC to advance their own interests. Because the typical MEC was composed of officers and department chairs, clinical sections began to clamor for departmental status. Today, it is common to see medical staffs with 10 to 15 departments, and some institutions have two to three times this many.

From relatively simple and straightforward organizations, medical staffs have morphed into large bureaucratic entities that require considerable support staff and make heavy demands on physicians' valuable and limited time. The list of responsibilities that department chairs must fulfill is imposing, perhaps made even more so considering that Joint Commission surveyors can challenge department chairs to demonstrate how they meet each one of those responsibilities as listed in MS.01.01.01 EP 36.

It is noted that departments are not required by TJC or HFAP. However, if your medical staff is organized into departments, it must meet certain requirements to comply. DNV has no regulatory standards for departments.

Clinical departments usually have their own policies and procedures—and even an array of officers to organize their activities and comply with these requirements. All of this requires time, effort, and expertise on the part of physicians to administer effectively. In addition, an increasing number of external parties (e.g., department of health, regulators, Office of Inspector General) are scrutinizing the work performed by the organized medical staff to ensure that important functions are not simply given lip service. If a clinical department is responsible for peer review, it must do more than simply go through the motions. Many clinical departments are looking for less burdensome ways to fulfill their responsibilities more effectively. Physicians have less time than ever to devote to medical staff citizenship responsibilities, especially as many are spending less time at the hospital to grow their private practices or pursue other professional activities. Many medical staffs have found that their work is best accomplished by a small cadre of well-trained leaders who can represent the broad interests of physicians and carry out medical staff work efficiently. Downsizing the medical staff bureaucratic structure facilitates this kind of transformation and, as a result, many medical staffs are consolidating their departments, with no detriment to the staff's ability to carry out critical functions. The federal government and accrediting bodies do not require the medical staff to be organized around departments, as long as it accomplishes its delegated functions. However, if a medical staff has departments, then each one must meet all of the requirements per the standards of the individual accreditation agency.

Whether the medical staff is organized into departments or not, many medical staffs have centralized the core functions and may simply carry out their critical work through key committees (e.g., the MEC, credentials committee, and peer review/quality committee). These committees can call on subject-matter experts from other departments' staff as necessary to facilitate initiatives.

As mentioned previously, reducing the number of departments or abolishing departments altogether often leads medical staffs to become concerned about maintaining adequate representation on the MEC. Changes in departmental configuration raise questions about which individuals will serve on the MEC, but there is no reason that the composition of the MEC must be tied to departmental structures (refer to the discussion earlier in this section about which individuals should be on the MEC).

The bottom line is that medical staffs are free to select from various organizational arrangements, and they should thoughtfully consider their options. Choose a medical staff structure that maximizes effectiveness and minimizes the burden on physicians' time. Given the challenges posed by our evolving healthcare system, medical staffs should not assume that a bureaucratic structure that served well in the past will remain the best choice going forward.

## Conflict Resolution

Most bylaws that I review contain a conflict resolution mechanism for when issues need to be addressed between the MEC and the board. This conflict resolution mechanism is usually a committee comprised of an equal number of individuals from both bodies, usually called the Joint Conference Committee.

If your hospital is Joint Commission– accredited, your medical staff must establish a new conflict resolution mechanism to comply with MS. 01.01.01, and it must be written into your bylaws. This conflict resolution mechanism must address conflict between the MEC and the organized medical staff. It can be as simple as a meeting between the officers of the medical staff and an equal number of concerned medical staff members. The conflict resolution mechanism could involve invoking the membership rights, as noted earlier. You may also use bylaws language as a guide to implement a conflict resolution mechanism.

### SAMPLE BYLAWS LANGUAGE

#### Conflict resolution between the medical staff and the MEC

Each staff member in the active category may challenge any rule, regulation, policy, or procedure established by the MEC through the following process:

1. The staff member submits to the [president of the medical staff/chief of staff] his or her challenge to the rule or policy in writing, including any recommended changes to the rule or policy.

2. At the MEC meeting that follows such notification, the MEC shall discuss the challenge and determine if it will change the rule or policy.

3. If changes are adopted, they will be communicated to the medical staff. At such time, each medical staff member in the active category may submit written notification of any further challenge(s) to the rule or policy to the [president of the medical staff/chief of staff].

4. In response to a written challenge to a rule or policy, the MEC may, but is not required to, appoint a task force to review the challenge and recommend potential changes to address concerns raised by the challenge.

  

## SAMPLE BYLAWS LANGUAGE

### Conflict resolution between the medical staff and the MEC (cont.)

5. If a task force is appointed, the MEC will take final action on the rule or policy based on the recommendations of the task force.

6. Once the MEC has taken final action in response to the challenge, with or without recommendations from a task force, any medical staff member may submit a petition signed by [X%] of the members of the active category requesting review and possible change of a rule, regulation, policy, or procedure. After receiving a petition, the MEC will follow the adoption procedure outlined in Section [X].

Each staff member in the active category may challenge any rule, regulation, policy,

If the medical staff votes to recommend directly to the board an amendment to the bylaws, rules or regulations, or policies that is different from what the MEC has recommended, the following conflict resolution process shall be followed:

- The MEC shall have the option of appointing a task force to review the differing recommendations of the MEC and the medical staff and recommend language to the bylaws, rules and regulations, or policies that is agreeable to both the medical staff and the MEC.

- Regardless of whether the MEC adopts modified language, the medical staff shall have the opportunity to recommend alternative language directly to the board. If the board receives differing recommendations for bylaws, rules and regulations, or policies from the MEC and the medical staff, the board shall have the option of appointing a task force to study the basis of the differing recommendations and to recommend appropriate board action.

- Regardless of whether the board appoints such a task force, the board shall have final authority to resolve the differences between the medical staff and the MEC. At any point in the process of addressing a disagreement between the medical staff and MEC regarding the bylaws, rules and regulations, or policies, the medical staff, MEC, or governing board shall each have the right to recommend using an outside facilitator to assist in addressing the disagreement. The final decision regarding whether to use an outside resource and the process that will be followed in so doing is the responsibility of the board.

  

## Amending the Bylaws

For many reasons, medical staffs have felt that getting bylaws endorsed or amended is more painful than a root canal. Most medical staff members have little interest in the details of bylaws language or the issues underlying certain bylaws. Medical staff apathy is widespread, and the specific details of medical staff functions addressed in the bylaws rarely seem of consequence, except to a few members. In addition, medical staff leaders often fail to adequately communicate to the staff the nature of the bylaws changes and the reasons behind the changes. As a result, many medical staffs have asked, "Is it necessary for the entire medical staff to vote every time we wish to change bylaws that address a credentialing requirement or a committee structure? Can the medical staff function as a representative democracy in which leaders can authorize changes in policies and procedures?"

In an attempt to streamline the amendment process and move to a more representative democracy, many medical staffs have divided their governing documents into the following:

- A core set of bylaws that rarely change
- Associated manuals that collate policies of similar content (e.g., a credentials manual, corrective action/fair hearing manual, organization and function manual)
- Additional medical staff policies, rules, and regulations

If governing documents are so divided, a practical and functional approach might require a general staff vote to modify only the bylaws. Informed medical staff leaders (e.g., the MEC) would be allowed to change the rules, regulations, or policies if delegated to do so by the medical staff. MS.01.01.01, mandates that core items (e.g., the credentialing process and fair hearing and appeal process) be outlined in the bylaws and then the associated documents (e.g., manuals, rules, regulations, or policies) can give the detail of the procedures. In other words, the bylaws can delineate the main header items with a brief one- or two-sentence explanation, and the remainder can reside in the associated documents. Many medical staffs have long handled their governing documents and related policies and procedures in this practical and efficient manner.

  

However, some physicians believe strongly that the general medical staff should be required to vote on all matters regarding the organization and structure of the medical staff, membership, credentialing and privileging, corrective action, and so forth. Although the regulatory agencies mandate that the medical staff adopt and amend the bylaws, the amount of detail regarding the credentialing and the fair hearing and appeal processes that will be placed in the bylaws (rather than associated documents) is up to individual medical staffs. The amount of detail in the bylaws is also partially determined by how burdensome the bylaws adoption and amendment process is; the more burdensome the process, the more detail is usually in associated documents. Some medical staffs choose to have all material in the bylaws because their amendment process is streamlined.

The confusing language in MS.01.01.01, which attempts to distinguish between "processes" and "procedural details," is ambiguous. This standard requires medical staffs to put all major substantive provisions in their medical staff bylaws. If a medical staff previously streamlined its governance documents into separate manuals (e.g., a credentials manual, organization and functions manual, or credentialing/privileging policies), one method to address MS.01.01.01 would be to rename all the documents as parts of the medical staff bylaws and then ask the entire medical staff to vote on them. A second method would be to keep the associated documents as is and only include vital aspects of the various processes in the bylaws.
For those hospitals accredited by TJC, MS.01.01.01 emphasizes that the medical staff has ultimate authority and votes on what authority it wants to delegate to the MEC. However, the medical staff cannot delegate the responsibility of bylaws adoption and amendment to the MEC. The medical staff must have the right to propose bylaws amendments directly to the board without going through the MEC. This offers a check-and-balance system so that issues that are important to a significant number of medical staff members cannot be stifled by the MEC's actions.

The medical staff can still delegate to the MEC the ability to enact rules, regulations, and policies. Just as with the bylaws, there needs to be a mechanism for the medical staff to also propose or reject rules, regulations, or policies if there is a significant concern. Any rules, regulations, or policies proposed by one party (the medical staff or MEC) must be communicated to the other party prior to a vote so that all actions are transparent. This check-and-balance system ensures that when issues arise that are of concern to a significant number of medical staff members, the MEC will address them.

Many medical staffs may want to reconsider the entire amendment process. If a medical staff wishes to amend a bylaw, most bylaws provisions require a two-thirds vote at a medical staff meeting (i.e., a quorum is met). Sometimes, the amendment cannot be adopted until the proposed changes have been read at multiple meetings. Although bylaws changes are custom arily brought to the staff for consideration after they have been vetted and recommended by the bylaws committee/MEC (although this is no longer the sole method per MS.01.01.01),

## SAMPLE BYLAWS LANGUAGE

### Amending the bylaws: Amendment, initiation, and communication

- Proposed amendments to these bylaws may originate from the MEC or a petition signed by [X%] of the voting members of the medical staff.
- When the MEC proposes changes and before it votes, it will communicate its proposed amendment to the medical staff.
- When the medical staff proposes changes and before it votes, it will communicate the proposed amendment to the MEC.
- Proposed amendments to these rules and regulations may originate from the MEC or by a petition signed by [X%] of the voting members of the medical staff.
- If the MEC does not pass the proposed amendment to the rules and regulations, the organized medical staff can ask for a medical staff vote using the mechanisms noted in the conflict resolution process.
- When the MEC adopts a policy or amendment thereto, it will communicate the amendment to the organized medical staff.

  

there always seem to be a few medical staff members who are disenchanted with the proposed changes. They distrust the motives of medical staff leaders who have studied the issues underlying the proposed changes and who are suggesting new bylaws language. Many times, the slightest dissent seems to stymie the ability of the medical staff to act.

Many staffs have implemented innovative approaches to bylaws amendments that they find more practical and flexible. When determining what your bylaws should allow, consider the following questions:

- Which individuals can recommend a bylaws amendment?
- Should an amendment vote occur at a meeting, or can it occur via mail-in ballots?
- What voting thresholds are needed for an amendment to pass, and how should the votes be counted?

Let's look more closely at each of these questions.

### *Which individuals can recommend a bylaws amendment?*

Medical staffs would not want to see any one individual force a proposed bylaws amendment through the voting process because this could jam up the medical staff and board with amendments that don't have signifcant support. In the past, any individual could propose an amendment, which was then vetted by a bylaws committee or the MEC. Under the new standard, this vetting process can be used, but it is no longer necessary. Rather, the medical staff can define when there is sufficient support for an amendment to go forward. The number should not be so low that only a handful of members can force a vote, thus causing a logjam of potential amendments. Conversely, the number should not be so high as to prohibit any medical staff–generated amendment proposal from going forward. It is recommended (and I feel this is in compliance with the intent of MS.01.01.01) that 25%–50% of the medical staff sign a petition before an amendment can go through the voting process.

## SAMPLE BYLAWS LANGUAGE

### Amending the bylaws: Review, revision, adoption, and amendment

The medical staff shall be responsible for formulating, reviewing (at least biennially), and recommending any medical staff bylaws, rules, regulations, policies, procedures, and amendments to the board as needed. These bylaws, rules, regulations, policies, procedures, and amendments shall be effective when approved by the board. The medical staff can exercise this responsibility through its elected and appointed leaders or through direct vote of its membership.

#### Methods of adoption and amendment to bylaws

Proposed amendments to bylaws may be originated by the MEC or by a petition signed by [X%] of the members of the active category. Each active member of the medical staff will be eligible to vote on the proposed amendment via a printed or secure electronic ballot in a manner determined by the MEC. All active members of the medical staff shall receive at least [X] days advance notice of the proposed changes. The following is to be adopted:

- [Option 1: The medical staff receives a simple majority (50% plus one), 66% (two-thirds), or 75% (three-fourths) vote cast by those active members eligible to vote on adoption and amendment.]
- [Option 2: The medical staff receives an affirmative vote by a simple majority, 66%, or 75% of those members eligible to vote. An affirmative vote will be counted by returning the ballot marked "yes," or by not returning the ballot.]
- [Option 3: The medical staff receives a return ballot marked "no" by 25%, 34%, or 50% of those members eligible to vote.]

Amendments so adopted shall be effective when approved by the board.

#### Methods of adoption and amendment to any medical staff rules, regulations, and policies

The medical staff may adopt additional rules, regulations, and policies as necessary to carry out its functions and meet its responsibilities under these bylaws. A rules and regulations manual and a policies manual may be used to organize these additional documents. The organized medical staff may delegate this responsibility to the MEC.

## SAMPLE BYLAWS LANGUAGE

### Amending the bylaws: Review, revision, adoption, and amendment (cont.)

Proposed amendments to the rules and regulations manual, and policies manual may be originated by the MEC. The MEC will communicate the proposed amendment to the organized medical staff prior to a vote.

The MEC shall vote on the proposed language changes at a regular meeting, or at a special meeting called for such purpose. Following an affirmative vote by the MEC, any of these documents may be adopted, amended, or repealed, in whole or in part, and such changes shall be effective when approved by the board.

In addition to the process described in [section on amendment process], the organized medical staff may recommend amendments to any rules, regulations, or policies directly to the board by submitting a petition signed by [X%] of the members of the active category. On presentation of such petition, the adoption process outlined in [section on amendment process] will be followed.

The MEC may adopt such amendments to these bylaws, rules, regulations, and policies that are, in the committee's judgment, technical or legal modifications or clarifications. Such modifications may include reorganization or renumbering, punctuation, spelling, or other errors of grammar or expression. Such amendments need not be approved by the entire board but must be approved by the hospital CEO. Neither the organized medical staff nor the board may unilaterally amend the medical staff bylaws or rules and regulations.

If the organized medical staff does not delegate the responsibility of adopting and amending medical staff rules or regulations, The Joint Commission allows that the MEC can enact rules and regulations that are necessary for legal or regulatory compliance after receiving approval by the board (MS.01.01.01 EP 11).

The MEC and the board may adopt such provisional amendments to these rules and regulations that they deem necessary for legal or regulatory compliance. After

  

SAMPLE BYLAWS LANGUAGE

**Amending the bylaws: Review, revision, adoption, and amendment (cont.)**

adoption, the MEC will communicate these provisional amendments to the rules and regulations to the organized medical staff for its review.

If the medical staff approves of the provisional amendment, the amendment will stand.

If the medical staff does not approve of the provisional amendment, this will be resolved using the conflict resolution mechanism noted in Section [X]. If a substitute amendment is then proposed, it will follow the usual approval process.

### *Should an amendment vote occur at a meeting, or can it occur via mail-in ballots?*

Most staffs have traditionally held bylaws amendment votes at general or special medical staff meetings. Because many physicians fail to attend meetings, and therefore fail to meet quorum requirements, many medical staffs have moved to a mail ballot approach. Some medical staffs have recognized that although mail ballots might be more convenient for physicians, many physicians fail to return their ballots. As noted previously, these staffs are now permitting physicians to vote electronically (via email or on a website), via fax ballot, or even over the phone. This provides all eligible voters the chance to vote.

### *What voting thresholds are needed for an amendment to pass?*

Requiring a simple majority (i.e., 50% plus one), two-thirds, or three-quarters affirmative vote are traditional options. Some medical staffs now use a mail or electronic ballot that lists the proposed changes and states that a staff member who does not return the ballot within the required time frame is presumed to have cast an affirmative vote. The premise is that if you fail to vote, you have indicated trust in your elected leaders to make proper decisions. An alternative is to state that no action is required to vote yes and that the ballot need only be returned if the medical staff member wishes to vote no. Although positive affirmation of a vote is preferable, voting members may not vote for various reasons, and voting quorums or thresholds may not be achieved. Some medical staffs have found the passive method of voting to work well. Consider the comment cards at a restaurant. If the meal is good and meets your expectations, you are not likely to fill out a comment card. However, if you are displeased with a meal, then you are more likely to fill out the comment card (or talk to the manager). When it comes to medical staffs, those who are displeased with an amendment are more likely to vote than those who are either pleased or are apathetic. Thus, the two-thirds approval rate can be measured by a one-third disapproval rate. Unless at least one-third of the voting members return a ballot voting "no," the amendment passes.

Many permutations can be drafted into the bylaws, but when choosing an approach, it is wise to consider the downside of gridlock when it comes to passing needed bylaws changes.

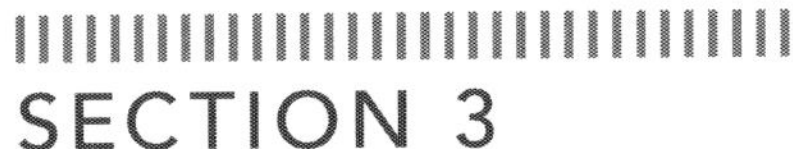

SECTION 3

# Member Rights, Corrective Action, and Fair Hearings

One of the most important functions of the bylaws is to state the rights and protections that are afforded to members of the medical staff. Because these rights and protections are often invoked under contentious circumstances that could lead to litigation, they need to be described in the bylaws clearly and meticulously. Sections of bylaws that address member rights, corrective action, and fair hearings also need to comply carefully with federal and state statutes and regulations, as well as accreditation standards.

The most important federal regulation to consider when drafting bylaws language regarding corrective action and fair hearings is the Health Care Quality Improvement Act of 1986 (HCQIA), which provides federal immunity from monetary damages for medical staff professional review actions. The definition of "professional review action" is found in HCQIA at 42 *USC* §11151(a) and reads as follows:

*The term "professional review action" means an action or recommendation of a professional review body that is taken or made in the conduct of professional review activity, which is based on the competence or professional conduct of an individual physician (which conduct affects or could affect adversely the health or welfare of a patient or patients), and which affects (or may affect) adversely the clinical privileges, or membership in a professional society, of the physician. Such term includes a formal decision of a professional review body not to take an action or make a recommendation described in the previous sentence and also includes professional review activities relating to a professional review action. In this section, an action is not considered to be based on the competence or professional conduct of a physician if the action is primarily based on the following:*

- *The physician's association, or lack of association, with a professional review society or association*

- *The physician's fees or the physician's advertising or engaging in other competitive acts intended to solicit or retain business*
- *The physician's participation in prepaid group health plans, salaried employment, or any other manner of delivering health services, whether on a fee-for-service or other basis*
- *The physician's association with, supervision of, delegation of authority to, support for, training of, or participation in a private group practice with a member or members of a particular class of healthcare practitioner or professional*
- *Any other matter that does not relate to the competence or professional conduct of a physician*

This statute prompted the creation of the federal National Practitioner Data Bank (NPDB) and its reporting requirements. HCQIA enumerates the elements and processes that medical staffs must make available to physicians undergoing corrective action. Many of these details are reviewed in this section.

A medical staff that takes action against a physician or dentist may be required to file a report with the NPDB. Because these reports can have a harmful effect on a practitioner's livelihood, it is important to understand when such reports should and should not be submitted. Carefully drafted bylaws can provide some clarity in this regard.

The government publishes a guidebook to the NPDB that is an excellent resource to consider when fashioning corrective action policies. The guidebook is currently being updated. This document can be located on the Internet at *www.npdb-hipdb.hrsa.gov/resources/NPDB-guidebook.pdf.*

In addition to HCQIA, every state has laws that affect the corrective action section of the medical staff bylaws. These include state peer review statutes and additional reporting regulations issued by state health departments or other government entities. When composing bylaws, it is always prudent to run the proposed changes by an attorney familiar with state law.

  

When creating text for medical staff corrective actions, keep three goals firmly in mind:

- The process must make patient safety and well-being the foremost consideration. The corrective action process should not be so onerous or convoluted that this goal is not readily achieved.

- The process must protect individual members of the medical staff from abuse by colleagues or hospital officials.

- The process should facilitate appropriate participation by members of the medical staff and protect them from retaliation by angry colleagues.

With regard to the final point, many medical staff bylaws detail the circumstances under which the hospital will indemnify medical staff members who are sued or dragged into litigation by a colleague. The bylaws should also clearly indicate that the medical staff peer review process and corrective actions recommended or taken by the medical staff and the board are intended to be fully protected by state and federal laws.

## Member Rights

The most fundamental rights granted to members of the medical staff relate to the process they are provided if the medical executive committee (MEC) recommends that corrective action is necessary. Corrective action is defined as the termination of medical staff membership or a restriction, reduction, modification, or termination of medical staff privileges for reasons of clinical incompetence or unprofessional conduct. For more on member rights, see Section 2.

## Collegial Intervention

Although we think medical staff leaders have the inherent authority to engage in collegial intervention, sometimes formal investigations are instituted solely because "that's what the bylaws require." Bylaws should allow medical staff leaders to address questions relating to an individual's clinical practice/professional conduct early and in a nonpunitive way so that "discipline" (and the negative effects of adverse actions) can be a last resort. The goal of these progressive steps, beginning with collegial and educational efforts, is to help the individual voluntarily respond to and resolve questions that have been raised. All collegial intervention efforts made by medical staff leaders and hospital management should be part of the performance improvement and professional and peer review activities of the hospital and medical staff. Collegial intervention efforts should be encouraged (but not mandatory) and should be within the discretion of the appropriate medical staff leaders and hospital management.

Collegial intervention efforts could involve any of the following activities:

- Educating and advising colleagues of all applicable policies, including those related to appropriate behavior, emergency call obligations, and the timely and adequate completion of medical records

- Following up on any questions or concerns raised about the clinical practice/conduct of privileged practitioners and recommending such steps as proctoring, monitoring, consultation, and letters of guidance

- Sharing summary comparative quality, utilization, and other relevant data to help individuals conform their practices to appropriate norms

If it appears that patients may be placed in harm's way while collegial interventions are undertaken or following collegial intervention efforts, if it appears that the practitioner's performance places patients in danger or compromises quality of care, the MEC will consider whether it should recommend to the board that the practitioner's membership/privileges be restricted or revoked. Before issuing such a recommendation, the MEC may authorize an investigation to determine whether sufficient evidence exists to support such a recommendation.

  

## Investigations

When the MEC suspects that there is reason to recommend corrective action against a medical staff member, it may first conduct an investigation into whether such a recommendation is warranted. Many medical staffs do not adequately differentiate between everyday peer review and a formal investigation. The latter typically follows peer review and is the process by which the MEC confirms that it has sufficient evidence to justify a recommendation for termination or restriction of privileges. On some occasions, the MEC may believe the evidence is so clear that an investigation is unnecessary. However, in most cases, it is prudent for an official investigation to precede a recommendation for corrective action.

As mentioned in Section 1, it is important to have a clear definition of "investigation" in your bylaws, because a failure to do so could have serious implications when reporting physicians to the NPDB. The NPDB requires hospitals to report practitioners who voluntarily surrender membership or clinical privileges while under investigation for possible clinical incompetence or unprofessional conduct. Therefore, if the medical staff reviews a physician's performance but mistakenly labels its actions an "investigation," the medical staff must report the physician to the NPDB, which could unnecessarily scar the physician's career.

The NPDB also requires hospitals to report physicians who surrender membership or clinical privileges in return for the hospital not conducting an investigation or taking a professional review action. The NPDB requires a report even when the practitioner is unaware of the investigation. A practitioner who surrenders membership or privileges while under investigation must be reported regardless of his or her stated reason (e.g., personal health concerns, retirement, relocation, or personal circumstances, such as divorce).

The NPDB guidebook states the following concerning investigations:

- An investigation should be carried out by the healthcare entity (e.g., the medical staff peer review committee) and not by an individual on the staff
- The hospital should create contemporaneous evidence of an ongoing investigation (e.g.,

meeting minutes, an order from a hospital leader initiating an investigation, letters to the practitioner involved)

- An investigation should address concerns about professional competence or conduct
- An investigation is considered ongoing until a final action is taken or it is formally closed
- An investigation should be a precursor to a professional review action
- A general or routine review of cases is not an investigation
- A general or routine review of a particular practitioner is not an investigation

A hospital should never make an improper report to the NPDB. A report made incorrectly can have a negative effect on a physician's career and can lead to litigation. Therefore, medical staff bylaws should clearly define the following criteria:

- When an investigation begins
- Who can initiate or authorize an investigation
- What the grounds are for an investigation
- Who will carry out the investigation
- How the investigation will be documented
- What the obligations are for reporting a voluntary surrender or plea bargain by the practitioner under investigation

When clinical issues arise during the peer review process, a focused review of the practitioner may ensue. The Joint Commission (TJC) refers to focused professional practice evaluation (FPPE) as the activity that takes place when a hospital questions a currently privileged practitioner's ability to provide safe, quality care. It is also defined as the process of confirming that a practitioner who is new to the medical staff is competent to carry out his or her privileges. Under the first definition of FPPE, the medical staff generally would not engage in a formal investigation. Competency evaluations are mandated by all accreditation agencies, including TJC, Det Norske Veritas, and the Healthcare Facilities Accreditation Program. The important thing to remember is that routine peer review, or any review focused on an individual, is still peer review. Only the MEC should decide when an investigation begins because doing so will help differentiate a formal investigation from peer review.

  

It is often most practical for the MEC to assign the duty of conducting investigations to an ad hoc investigation committee. This committee should be responsible for looking into the available evidence and making an initial recommendation regarding the need for corrective action. The bylaws should specify how this committee is composed and how members are appointed.

When appointing members for the investigation committee, fundamental conflict-of-interest policies should be considered. Also, it is generally wise to avoid assigning partners or associates of the physician under review. Likewise—to the degree feasible when the medical staff is small—physicians who are in significant referral relationships or who are significant economic competitors of the physician under investigation should not be appointed to the investigating body.

However, HCQIA and some hospital bylaws do not expressly preclude direct economic competitors from participating in investigations. Although it is wise to not have direct economic competitors on the investigative body, the option to not preclude direct economic competitors is in place so should litigation arise, there is no second-guessing over whether the individuals on the committee were significant economic competitors and therefore placed on the investigating committee in violation of the bylaws. When composing an investigating committee, it is also prudent to check your state's peer review laws. A few states have laws outlining the parameters for assigning individuals to an investigating committee.

The governing documents may also address whether hospitals are permitted to use outside consultants to help the committee interpret evidence unearthed during an investigation, or to provide external peer review of charts or cases. The documents should indicate which leaders could authorize the use of an external peer reviewer. Generally, these documents should make it clear that the physician under review does not have the right to compel the medical staff to perform an external review.

It is important that the investigation be conducted in a manner perceived as fair to the practitioner involved. Therefore, bylaws should state:

- Any requirement the medical staff has to notify the practitioner when an investigation is initiated
- The process by which the practitioner under investigation may provide information to the investigating committee
- The fact that the practitioner has no right to legal representation when he or she is brought before the investigating committee, because this is an administrative rather than a legal proceeding

Volunteer leaders may understandably fear that they will be the targets of threats, intimidation, or litigation. In difficult situations involving disruptive physicians, it is perfectly acceptable to have the hospital governing board and management assume the lead role in the investigation. This is particularly true when no clinical issues are raised and, thus, clinical expertise is not needed. The bylaws should articulate this option if it is desired.

## SAMPLE BYLAWS LANGUAGE

### Investigations

#### Initiation

A request for an investigation must be submitted by a medical staff officer, committee chair, department chief, CEO, chief medical officer, or hospital board chair to the MEC. The request must be supported by references to the specific activities or conduct of concern. If the MEC accepts the request and initiates an investigation, it shall appropriately document its reasons.

#### Investigation

An investigation can only begin if the MEC decides that it is warranted via an affirmative vote. In the event the board believes the MEC has incorrectly determined that an investigation is unnecessary, it may direct the MEC to proceed with an investigation.

The MEC may conduct the investigation itself or may assign the task to an appropriate standing or ad hoc committee of the medical staff.

  

## SAMPLE BYLAWS LANGUAGE

### Investigations (cont.)

If the investigation is delegated to a committee other than the MEC, such committee shall proceed with the investigation promptly and forward a written report of its findings, conclusions, and recommendations to the MEC as soon as practicable. The committee conducting the investigation shall have the authority to review all documents it considers relevant; interview individuals; consider appropriate clinical literature and practice guidelines; and use the resources of an external consultant if deemed necessary and such action is approved by the MEC and the CEO.

The investigating body may also require the practitioner under review to undergo a physical and/or mental examination and may subsequently access the results of such exams. The investigating body shall notify the practitioner in question that the investigation is being conducted and give the practitioner an opportunity to provide information in a manner that the investigating body deems appropriate.

The meeting between the physician in question and the investigating body (and meetings with any other individuals the investigating body chooses to interview) shall not constitute a "hearing," as that term is used in the hearing and appeals sections of these bylaws. The procedural rules with respect to hearings or appeals shall not apply to these meetings either. The individual being investigated shall not have the right to be represented by legal counsel before the investigating body or to compel the medical staff to engage external consultation.

Despite the status of any investigation, the MEC shall retain the authority and discretion to take whatever action may be warranted by the circumstances, including suspension, termination of the investigative process, or other action.

## Special Meeting Attendance Requirements

It is not uncommon for practitioners to delay any potential adverse action by not participating in any meeting that focuses on these issues. Many medical staffs have found it useful to have a mandatory attendance requirement at significant meetings scheduled to discuss a practitioner's performance. Medical staffs should consider requiring in the bylaws a member's participation in any special meeting called to address the member's clinical performance or professional conduct. Such a provision ensures that medical staff leadership can communicate concerns to the practitioner and lay out any expectations they have for performance improvement. Unfortunately, practitioners who resent that others are overseeing their performance frequently ignore requests to have such conversations.

Whenever the medical staff suspects that a physician has deviated from standard clinical or professional practice, the practitioner may be required to meet with the president of the medical staff, appropriate committee chair, or the standing or ad hoc committee that is considering the matter. The individual or group that is looking into the physician's performance and conduct should give the physician notice of the meeting a specified number of days (typically five) prior to the meeting and notify the physician that his or her presence is mandatory. The medical staff may choose to automatically terminate the membership/privileges of any practitioner who fails to attend such a meeting after receiving two notices. Termination would not give rise to a fair hearing, but it would be automatically rescinded if and when the practitioner participates in the meeting.

## Suspensions

Suspensions are sometimes the end result of a corrective action process. Suspensions can also be invoked in advance of an investigation in which medical staff or hospital leaders perceive an immediate danger to patients. Suspensions are also used for administrative reasons, such as a physician's failure to maintain licensure or professional liability insurance or for failure to complete medical records.

Because suspensions are highly disruptive to a clinician's practice and can harm that individual's reputation, they should be invoked only when clearly necessary and always in strict compliance with the procedures described in the bylaws. When writing bylaws provisions that address suspensions, it is important to recognize that suspensions must be reported to the NPDB when they:

- Last for more than 30 days
- Are imposed because of a concern about professional incompetence or unprofessional conduct
- Result from a professional review action by the hospital

If a physician or dentist resigns while under suspension for reasons of competence or conduct, the event must be reported to the NPDB, as would any surrender of privileges while under investigation. It is also important to recognize that the HCQIA considers summary suspensions to be a professional review action and, if imposed for more than 14 days, should entitle the suspended clinician to hearing and appeals rights. Failure to grant these rights to the physician may make the professional review body ineligible for the immunity protections provided by HCQIA.

It is common for medical staff bylaws to describe various types of suspensions, including regular disciplinary, automatic, and summary/precautionary suspensions. The following paragraphs will discuss various approaches that reflect this diverse terminology.

### *Summary/precautionary suspensions*

The term "summary suspension" generally refers to a suspension of some or all of a practitioner's privileges based on the medical staff's determination that allowing the practitioner to continue without such limitation would put patients in harm's way. Many hospitals have adopted the term "precautionary suspension" to better reflect the nature of a suspension that is imposed when patient safety is a concern. Both terms are interchangeable and are acceptable to use in the bylaws.

The bylaws should specify which individuals and committees can impose a summary suspension and state what access the suspended practitioner will have to a hearing and appeal. If a summary/precautionary suspension imposed for reasons of competence or conduct lasts more than 14 days, the practitioner must have access to the fair hearing and appeal process.

### *Automatic suspensions and relinquishments*

Bylaws typically articulate the circumstances under which the medical staff will automatically suspend a practitioner's privileges because of his or her failure to comply with one or more administrative requirements. These suspensions usually conclude once the practitioner complies with the requirement(s). Because these suspensions do not reflect a judgment on the practitioner's competence or professional conduct, they do not typically entitle the practitioner to a hearing or appeal, and they are not reportable to the NPDB. State statutes may require reporting above and beyond the requirements of the NPDB, so review your state's laws before writing this bylaws language.

Many hospitals have replaced the term "automatic suspension" with "automatic relinquishment," wherein practitioners lose their privileges because they did not adhere to basic rules established in the bylaws or they failed to meet requirements mandated by state laws or regulations. Relinquishment can also be applied to situations in which the state board or another entity has taken action against a practitioner's licensure status.

In these circumstances, there is no need for a hearing because the relinquishment is not a result of the hospital's determination that the practitioner is incompetent or has engaged in unprofessional conduct. It is the practitioner's failure to maintain eligibility for membership that triggered the automatic suspension or relinquishment; thus, the practitioner—not the hospital—is responsible for the consequences.

SAMPLE BYLAWS LANGUAGE

**Automatic relinquishment**

In the following circumstances, the practitioner's privileges and/or membership will be considered relinquished or limited as described, and the action shall be final without a right to hearing. If the physician disputes that these circumstances have occurred, the relinquishment, suspension, or limitation will stand until the MEC determines whether it is applicable. The MEC will make such a determination as soon as is practicable. The

SAMPLE BYLAWS LANGUAGE

## Automatic relinquishment (cont.)

president of the medical staff may reinstate the practitioner's privileges or membership after determining that the triggering circumstances have been rectified or no longer exist within 60 days of the relinquishment. After 60 days, the practitioner must reapply for membership and/or privileges. In addition, further corrective action may be recommended in accordance with these bylaws whenever any of the following actions occur:

### Licensure

**Revocation and suspension:** Whenever a practitioner's license or other legal credential authorizing him or her to practice in this state is revoked, suspended, expired, or voluntarily relinquished, the practitioner will automatically relinquish his or her medical staff membership and clinical privileges as of the date such action becomes effective.

**Restriction:** Whenever a practitioner's license or other legal credential authorizing him or her to practice is limited or restricted by an applicable licensing or certifying authority, any clinical privileges that the practitioner has been granted at this hospital that are within the scope of said limitation or restriction shall be automatically limited or restricted in a similar manner, as of the date such action becomes effective and throughout its term.

**Probation:** Whenever a practitioner is placed on probation by the applicable licensing or certifying authority, his or her membership status and clinical privileges shall automatically become subject to the same terms and conditions of the probation as of the date such action becomes effective and throughout its term.

**Medicare, Medicaid, Tricare, or other federal programs:** Whenever a practitioner is barred from Medicare, Medicaid, Tricare, or other federal programs, medical staff membership and clinical privileges shall be considered automatically relinquished as of the date such action becomes effective. Any practitioner listed on the U.S. Department of Health and Human Services Office of the Inspector General's list of excluded individuals/entities will be considered to have automatically relinquished his or her privileges.

SAMPLE BYLAWS LANGUAGE

## Automatic relinquishment (cont.)

### Controlled substances

**Drug Enforcement Agency certificate:** Whenever a practitioner's U.S. Drug Enforcement Agency (DEA) certificate or state-controlled substance registration (if applicable) is revoked, limited, or suspended, the practitioner will automatically and correspondingly be divested of the right to prescribe medications covered by the certificate, as of the date such action becomes effective and throughout its term.

**Probation:** Whenever a practitioner's DEA certificate or state-controlled substance registration (if applicable) is subject to probation, the practitioner's right to prescribe such medications shall automatically become subject to the same terms of the probation, as of the date such action becomes effective and throughout its term.

### Medical record completion requirements

A practitioner will be considered to have voluntarily relinquished the privilege to admit new patients or schedule new procedures whenever he or she fails to complete medical records within time frames established by the MEC. This relinquishment of privileges shall not apply to patients admitted or already scheduled at the time of relinquishment, to emergency patients, or to imminent deliveries. The relinquished privileges will be automatically restored when the medical records are completed in compliance with medical records policies.

### Professional liability insurance

Failure of a practitioner to maintain professional liability insurance in the amount required by state regulations and medical staff and board policies, and sufficient to cover the clinical privileges granted, shall result in immediate automatic relinquishment of a practitioner's clinical privileges. If, within 60 calendar days of the relinquishment, the practitioner does not provide evidence of required professional liability insurance (including coverage for any period during which insurance was not maintained), the

  

SAMPLE BYLAWS LANGUAGE

## Automatic relinquishment (cont.)

practitioner shall not be considered for reinstatement and shall be considered to have voluntarily resigned from the medical staff. The practitioner must notify the medical staff services department immediately of any change in professional liability insurance carrier or coverage.

### Medical staff dues and special assessments

Failure to promptly pay medical staff dues or any special assessment shall be considered an automatic relinquishment of a practitioner's appointment. A practitioner who does not remit such payments within 60 calendar days of receiving written warning of the delinquency shall be considered to have voluntarily resigned membership on the medical staff.

### Felony conviction

A practitioner who has been convicted of, or pled "guilty" or "no contest" or its equivalent to a felony involving violence, physical or sexual abuse, drug offenses, or insurance/healthcare fraud or abuse in any jurisdiction shall automatically relinquish medical staff membership and privileges. Such relinquishment shall become effective immediately on such indictment, conviction, or plea, regardless of whether an appeal is filed. Such relinquishment shall remain in effect until the matter is resolved by subsequent action of the board or through corrective action, if necessary.

### Failure to satisfy the special appearance requirement

A practitioner who fails without good cause to appear at a meeting where a special appearance is required, in accordance with these bylaws, shall be considered to have automatically relinquished all clinical privileges with the exception of emergencies and imminent deliveries. These privileges will be restored when the practitioner complies with the special appearance requirement. Failure to comply within 30 calendar days will be considered a voluntary resignation from the medical staff.

SAMPLE BYLAWS LANGUAGE

## Automatic relinquishment (cont.)

### Failure to participate in an evaluation

A practitioner who fails to participate in an evaluation of his or her qualifications for medical staff membership or privileges as required under these bylaws (whether an evaluation of physical or mental health or of clinical management skills), shall be considered to have automatically relinquished all privileges. These privileges will be restored when the practitioner complies with the requirement for an evaluation. Failure to comply within 30 calendar days will be considered a voluntary resignation from the medical staff.

### Failure to become board certified or failure to maintain board certification, if applicable

A practitioner who fails to become board certified or maintain board certification, if applicable, in compliance with these bylaws or medical staff credentialing policies, will be deemed to have immediately and voluntarily relinquished his or her medical staff appointment and clinical privileges (unless an exception is granted by the board based on a recommendation from the MEC).

### Failure to execute release and/or provide documents

A practitioner who fails to execute a general or specific release and/or provide documents to the president of the medical staff or designee on request shall be considered to have automatically relinquished all privileges. These documents are to help the medical staff president or designee evaluate the competency and credentialing/privileging qualifications of the practitioner in question. If the release is executed and/or documents provided within 30 calendar days of the practitioner receiving the notice of the automatic relinquishment, the practitioner may be reinstated. Thereafter, the member will be deemed to have resigned voluntarily from the staff and must reapply for staff membership and privileges.

  

## The Medical Staff Fair Hearing

The process of a hearing following the MEC's recommendation for corrective action is an important right that must be spelled out in the bylaws. It is essential that this section of the bylaws is carefully thought out, drafted with precision, and in strict compliance with the minimum procedural process required under HCQIA for the medical staff to have the immunity protections of this act. Although the process that the medical staff offers does not need to be equivalent to that available in a court of law, it must be sufficient for courts to consider the proceeding fair.

It is equally important that the bylaws are clear whether the hearing procedures apply only to members of the medical staff or to all practitioners with privileges. Most hospitals articulate one hearing plan for physicians, dentists, and other members of the medical staff and another for privileged practitioners who are not members, such as allied health professionals. The fair hearing and appeal process for privileged practitioners who are not members, and not physicians or dentists, is provided in Section 5 of this book.

Let's examine the factors that trigger a fair hearing and—equally important—those that do not.

SAMPLE BYLAWS LANGUAGE

### Events that trigger an offer for a hearing

#### Initiation of hearing

A physician, dentist, or any practitioner eligible for medical staff appointment shall be entitled to request a hearing whenever the MEC or the board makes an unfavorable recommendation with regard to clinical competence or professional conduct. Hearings will be triggered only by the following actions when the basis for such action is related to clinical competence or professional conduct:

- Denial of medical staff appointment or reappointment
- Revocation of medical staff appointment

SAMPLE BYLAWS LANGUAGE

### Events that trigger an offer for a hearing (cont.)

- Denial or restriction of requested clinical privileges
- Involuntary reduction or revocation of clinical privileges
- Application of a mandatory concurring consultation requirement or an increase in the stringency of a preexisting mandatory concurring consultation requirement, when such requirement only applies to an individual medical staff member and is imposed for more than 14 calendar days
- Suspension of staff appointment or clinical privileges, but only if such suspension is for more than 14 calendar days and is not caused by the member's failure to complete medical records or any other reason unrelated to clinical competence or professional conduct

## *Events that do not trigger an offer for a hearing*

Any activity that does not deny, terminate, or restrict privileges for more than 14 days, and is done for a reason related to competence or conduct, does not invoke fair hearing and appeal rights. Some medical staffs have delineated a laundry list of these activities. The simplest language is " . . . any activity other than those that invoke fair hearing and appeal rights does not invoke the right to a fair hearing or appeal."

## *Loss of privileges consequent to an exclusive provider agreement*

If a practitioner loses privileges or membership because the hospital offers an exclusive contract to another practitioner or specialty group, a fair hearing is not triggered at most institutions and the action is not reported to the NPDB. Most hospitals have one or more exclusive contracts with members of the medical staff to ensure round-the-clock coverage for a particular service. Most institutions do not want to waste resources on fair hearings when they exclude physicians to comply with an exclusive contract. Nevertheless, physicians who find themselves ineligible to hold certain privileges as a result of an exclusive arrangement may sue the hospital. Courts generally analyze the hospital's medical staff bylaws and contracts to see if the language supports an interpretation that a hearing is required. Therefore, medical staff bylaws must address what hearing rights, if any, the hospital offers members who are affected by the initiation or ongoing existence of an exclusive contract.

Check your state laws before addressing this issue in your bylaws. Most state courts have supported hospitals that deny hearings in these circumstances because the exclusive contracts reflect the hospital's business decisions and not determinations of physician competence. Regardless of how you choose to handle this situation in your institution, it is wise to spell it out in your medical staff bylaws.

## SAMPLE BYLAWS LANGUAGE

### Exclusive contracts

Whenever hospital policy specifies that certain hospital facilities or services may be provided on an exclusive basis in accordance with contracts or letters of agreement between the hospital and qualified practitioners, other practitioners must, except in an emergency or life-threatening situation, adhere to the exclusivity policy when arranging for or providing care. Application for initial appointment or for clinical privileges related to the hospital facilities or services covered by exclusive agreements will not be accepted or processed unless submitted in accordance with the existing contract or agreement with the hospital. Practitioners who have previously been granted privileges, which now become covered by an exclusive contract, will not be able to exercise those privileges unless they become a party to the contract.

**Effect of contract or employment expiration or termination**

The effect of expiration or other termination of a contract on a practitioner's staff appointment and clinical privileges will be governed solely by the terms of the practitioner's contract with the hospital. If the contract or the employment agreement is silent on the matter, then contract expiration or other termination alone will not affect the practitioner's staff appointment status or clinical privileges.

## *Hearing procedural matters*

The medical staff bylaws should clearly articulate a member's right to a hearing, as well as how that hearing will be conducted. Although the hearing procedures are not required to provide the same procedural safeguards that courts of law do, certain minimum procedural standards must be met for the hearing process to be considered "fair" under HCQIA.

Often, the courts answer the question of whether a member has received adequate procedural protections by examining whether the hospital has complied with its own fair hearing procedures. Therefore, while ensuring fairness, the procedures should be written clearly and should not impose hurdles that are overly burdensome on the medical staff or institution. Important procedural issues to be addressed include the following:

- Notice of a hearing and the circumstances that trigger a hearing
- Waiver of a hearing
- Hearing participants
- Time frame for events surrounding a hearing (e.g., how many days the physician has to request a fair hearing after receiving notice of an adverse action, how many days the medical staff has to respond to the physician's request)
- The burden of proof that will be required
- The presentation and admissibility of evidence
- The role of attorneys

## *Waiver of right to a fair hearing*

Once the hospital offers a hearing to a medical staff member, it is up to that member to request the hearing. The bylaws should address the circumstances in which a practitioner waives the right to a hearing. HCQIA mandates that the affected practitioner has 30 days to formally request a fair hearing.

  

SAMPLE BYLAWS LANGUAGE

### Waiver of right to a fair hearing

In the event the affected individual does not request a hearing in the time and manner required by these bylaws, the individual shall be deemed to have waived the right to such hearing and to have accepted the recommendation made by the medical staff. Such recommended action shall become effective immediately on final board action.

## *Notice of a hearing*

Under HCQIA, if a physician requests a hearing on a timely basis, he or she must be given notice with the date, time, and location of the hearing. This date must not be sooner than 30 days after notice of the hearing is received by the practitioner (it can be shorter in cases of summary/precautionary suspension already in effect with the mutual agreement of all parties). The notice of the hearing must also contain a list of the witnesses, if any, expected to present at the hearing on behalf of the MEC and the hospital. Note: The practitioner can also call witnesses after giving notice, but it would not be in the notice of a hearing that the hospital/medical staff sends to the practitioner.

Note: Some states' statutes impose additional requirements for the notice of a hearing (e.g., a list of exhibits the MEC and the hospital expect to present). Check with state law to see what additional information you need to include in your bylaws.

## *Conduct of a hearing*

The two essential legal components of procedural fairness, as enumerated in HCQIA and articulated in most judicial decisions, are adequate notice and an opportunity to be heard before an impartial body. Thus, it is important for the bylaws to indicate which individuals may participate on a hearing panel, how they will be chosen, and who will choose them. Most hearings are contentious affairs and, when not conducted rigorously, can be unnecessarily long and confusing to the parties involved. As a result, it is critical for the medical staff to provide as much guidance as possible in the bylaws or hearing plan so that the proceedings can move forward under clear parameters.

## *Composition of the hearing panel*

There are several options for constructing a hearing panel. HCQIA states that, if requested on a timely basis, the hearing shall be held (as determined by the healthcare entity):

- Before an arbitrator who is mutually acceptable to the physician and the health-care entity
- Before a hearing officer who is appointed by the healthcare entity and who is not in direct economic competition with the physician involved
- Before a panel of individuals appointed by the healthcare entity who are not in direct economic competition with the physician

Arbitration is an option that is allowed by HCQIA, but my experience shows that few medical staffs follow this option. If an arbitration option is offered in the medical staff bylaws, secure the counsel of a knowledgeable healthcare attorney when drafting the appropriate clauses.

Most medical staffs prefer that a hearing panel—rather than a single hearing officer—hear corrective action disputes. However, a single hearing officer can be extremely helpful for some disputes. For example, on a small medical staff, it may be difficult to find eligible or willing practitioners to sit on a panel, and thus a single hearing officer is the best option for most cases being reviewed.

A hearing officer is sometimes preferred when the issue of dispute is one of professional conduct rather than clinical competence. The use of a hearing officer in lieu of a panel is less burdensome on the members of the medical staff, and the hearing is better facilitated when scheduling challenges, dialogue to accommodate, and complicated deliberations are all lessened. Often the hearing officer is a lawyer or retired judge—an individual with experience administering due process. The medical staff bylaws should clearly identify if, and under what circumstances, a hearing officer may be used.

If a panel is used, a hospital should call on individuals who are objective and free of personal bias or prejudice against the practitioner of concern. HCQIA states that members of the hearing panel cannot be in "direct economic competition" with the practitioner who has requested the hearing. It is also wise not to include the physician's practice partner or anyone the physician has a significant referral relationship with because such individuals may be biased. Your bylaws must articulate what constitutes these various relationships.

Medical staff bylaws should specify the requirements individuals must meet to serve on a hearing panel. However, they should not draw the parameters too narrowly because the hospital may subsequently find itself unable to fill positions on the panel. For example, it is wise not to strictly limit panel participation to active members of the medical staff or even to limit it to practitioners on the medical staff. Some medical staffs have practitioners from outside their hospital serve on hearing panels.

HCQIA allows the use of nonphysicians on a hearing panel. However, any time a hospital contemplates having a nonphysician on the panel, it should consult state law. The bylaws should also address whether physicians employed by or contracted with the hospital are eligible to serve on the hearing panel.

The bylaws should specify which individual(s) has the authority to appoint panel members. HCQIA states that panel selection is the hospital's responsibility. However, hearing panel selection is frequently a joint decision between the CEO and the president of the medical staff. If hospital administration delegates the responsibility of choosing hearing panel members to the medical staff, the bylaws should reflect this decision. The bylaws should also state whether there are any circumstances under which an individual can challenge the appointments made to the hearing panel.

The bylaws may also state whether the panel will be run by a member of the panel or by a presiding officer who runs the hearing process but is not a voting member of the panel. Many medical staffs find that a presiding officer, who is commonly a lawyer or retired judge knowledgeable about due process, relieves the physician members on the panel from interpreting and deciding on the legal questions and protocol to allow them to focus on the issue at hand. Some bylaws specifically require that the presiding officer or chairperson has no relationship with the hospital or the involved practitioner to avoid the perception of conflict of interest.

In some states, the local peer review statute may address the composition of a hearing panel. For example, several states require that hearing panels be made up of medical staff members. Your organization should check with local laws before finalizing this language in the medical staff bylaws.

As noted previously, there are certain circumstances in which a hearing officer, instead of a hearing panel, should be used. The CEO, acting for the board and after considering the recommendations of the medical staff president (or those of the chair of the board, if the hearing is the result of a board determination), may instead appoint a hearing officer to perform the functions that would otherwise be carried out by the hearing panel.

The hearing officer may not be any individual who is in direct economic competition with the individual requesting the hearing and shall not act as a prosecuting officer or as an advocate to either side at the hearing.

It is the choice of the hospital (usually in conjunction with the medical staff president) which fair hearing method to use in any particular case, as allowed by the medical staff bylaws. The practitioner whose actions initiated this hearing does not have the ability to choose the hearing method.

### *Pre-hearing conference*

The fair hearing plan in the bylaws should describe the processes for orchestrating and running a hearing. The more detail that can be provided, the less chance there is for controversy once a hearing is underway. The bylaws may also describe a pre-hearing conference. This is an opportunity for the hearing officer, presiding officer, or panel chair to meet with a representative of the involved practitioner and of the MEC (or the board, depending on who initiated the recommendation for corrective action) and establish the ground rules for the individuals who will present at the hearing. The physician's representative may be an attorney, a colleague, or even the practitioner, if he or she elects to self-represent. An effective pre-hearing conference should resolve all procedural questions, including any objections to exhibits or witnesses, and determine the time to be allotted to each testimony and cross-examination, thus preventing unnecessarily long hearings.

### *Burden of proof*

It is up to the medical staff to articulate the burden of proof that the hearing officer or panel will require to support or reject the MEC's or board's recommendation. For example, some bylaws require the practitioner who is the subject of the hearing to show that the MEC's recommendation is "arbitrary and capricious" or that it is not supported by "clear and convincing evidence." Others state that each side has an equal burden of proof and that the preponderance of evidence will prevail. HCQIA has published no mandate on the appropriate burden of proof that should be imposed at a hearing.

The decision regarding the appropriate burden of proof is again a cultural one. On one hand, the MEC (or board) has already done due diligence by making its recommendation for corrective action, and the hearing is considered an appeal of the initial decision. On the other hand, the hearing could be thought of as a completely new situation, and whichever side has the preponderance of the evidence prevails.

SAMPLE BYLAWS LANGUAGE

**Burden of proof**

The hearing panel shall recommend in favor of the MEC (or the board) unless it finds that the individual who requested the hearing has proved with a preponderance of the evidence that the recommendation that prompted the hearing was arbitrary, capricious, or appears to be unfounded or not supported by credible evidence. It is the burden of the practitioner under review to demonstrate that he or she satisfies, on a continuing basis, all criteria for initial appointment, reappointment, and clinical privileges, and fully complies with all medical staff and hospital policies.

### *Admissibility of evidence and requests for information or documents*

The bylaws or hearing plan (if the process is noted in the bylaws and the procedure is noted in a separate document) should make clear the following:

- What information may be entered into evidence
- What documents each side may request of the other
- What limits exist on the presentation of evidence

Both parties have the right to present evidence that the presiding officer determines is relevant regardless of its admissibility in a court of law. The presiding officer or panel chair should also have the ability to bar testimony that is irrelevant. It may be important to specifically state that peer review findings or records on other members of the medical staff are not considered relevant evidence and may not be introduced at the hearing. Some bylaws incorporate the "rule of relevance" approach used by courts.

All proposed exhibits must be provided to the other party by a predetermined time prior to the hearing. All objections to witnesses or documents should be submitted prior to the hearing.

SAMPLE BYLAWS LANGUAGE

**Provision of relevant information**

There is no right to formal "discovery" in connection with the hearing. The presiding officer, hearing panel chair, or hearing officer shall rule on any dispute regarding discoverability. This individual may impose safeguards, including denial or limitation of discovery, to protect the peer review process and ensure a reasonable and fair hearing. In general, the individual requesting the hearing shall be entitled on specific request, subject to a stipulation signed by both parties, the individual's counsel, and any experts that such documents shall be maintained as confidential consistent with all applicable state and federal peer review and privacy statutes and shall not be disclosed or used for any purpose outside of the hearing. These documents include the following:

- Copies of, or reasonable access to, all patient medical records referred to in the statement of reasons, at the practitioner's expense

SAMPLE BYLAWS LANGUAGE

**Provision of relevant information (cont.)**

- Reports of experts the MEC relied on
- Copies of redacted relevant committee minutes
- Copies of any other documents the MEC or board relied on

The practitioner in question is not entitled to the following:

- Information regarding other practitioners
- Evidence unrelated to the reasons for the recommendation or to the individual's qualifications for appointment or the relevant clinical privileges

### *Persons who may be present*

The bylaws should make clear which individuals may be present during a fair hearing. For example, the medical staff should determine whether the CEO, the medical staff president, or other administrative personnel may attend.

### *Scheduling*

The bylaws should describe how the hearing meetings will be scheduled and how postponements and extensions will be granted, as well as other matters of relevance to ensure that the hearing occurs in a timely fashion. Typically, the presiding officer has the discretion to set matters of schedule.

### *Role of attorneys*

HCQIA requires that the practitioner requesting the hearing has the right to representation by an attorney or other person of the practitioner's choice. However, the bylaws can specify restrictions on the role of legal counsel that, for example, prevent them from directly examining or cross-examining witnesses. The bylaws can also give the hearing panel chair or presiding officer latitude to make such determinations. HCQIA specifically says that a hospital does not need to offer all of the procedural protections that are described in other legal proceedings.

A common perception is that attorneys create an adversarial and contentious atmosphere at hearings. However, sometimes attorneys smooth the process because of their familiarity with procedures similar to those of fair hearings. Regardless of which path your medical staff takes, the bylaws should make clear whether practitioners who are the subject of a hearing may have their lawyers present their case, examine witnesses, or advocate for their position. Some medical staffs limit lawyers to providing counsel and guidance to their client, although others allow them into the hearing room but limit their participation to procedural matters only. In the latter case, examination and cross-examination of witnesses is typically left to the practitioner. Notably, certain states may have laws governing public hospitals' actions in this regard.

Any individuals requesting a hearing who do not testify on their own behalf may be called and examined as if under cross-examination. The hearing panel may also question the witnesses, call additional witnesses, or request additional documentary evidence.

### *Decision of the hearing panel*

The bylaws should describe the manner in which the hearing panel delivers its findings. The panel should issue a written report that addresses the issues for which the hearing was convened, and all members of the hearing panel should sign the final report. The decision must not only go to the organization but to the involved practitioner as well.

**SAMPLE BYLAWS LANGUAGE**

**Appeals to the board**

**Time for appeal**

Within 10 calendar days after the hearing panel makes a recommendation, either the practitioner subject to the hearing or the MEC may appeal the recommendation. The request for appellate review shall be in writing and shall be delivered to the CEO or designee either in person or by certified mail. The request shall include a brief statement of the reasons for appeal and the specific facts or circumstances that justify further review. If such appellate review is not requested within 10 calendar days, both parties shall be deemed to have accepted the recommendation, and the hearing panel's report and recommendation shall be forwarded to the board.

  

SAMPLE BYLAWS LANGUAGE

## Appeals to the board (cont.)

### Grounds for appeal

The grounds for appeal shall be limited to the following:

- One or more parties failed to comply with the medical staff bylaws prior to or during the hearing so as to deny a fair hearing
- The recommendation of the hearing panel was made arbitrarily, capriciously, or with prejudice
- The recommendation of the hearing panel was not supported by substantial evidence based on the hearing record

### Time, place, and notice

Whenever an appeal is requested as set forth in the preceding sections, the chair of the board shall schedule and arrange for an appellate review as soon as arrangements can be reasonably made, taking into account the schedules of all individuals involved. The affected individual shall be given notice of the time, place, and date of the appellate review. The chair of the board may extend the time for appellate review for good cause.

### Nature of appellate review

- The chair of the board shall appoint a review panel composed of at least three members of the board to consider the information on which the recommendation was made. Members of this review panel may not be direct competitors of the practitioner under review and should not have participated in any formal investigation leading to the recommendation for corrective action that is under consideration.
- The review panel may, but is not required to, accept additional oral or written evidence subject to the same procedural constraints in effect for the hearing panel or hearing officer. Such additional evidence shall be accepted only if the party seeking to admit it can demonstrate that it is new, relevant evidence, and that any opportunity to admit it at the hearing was denied.

  

SAMPLE BYLAWS LANGUAGE

## Appeals to the board (cont.)

- Each party shall have the right to present a written statement in support of its position on appeal. In its sole discretion, the review panel may allow each party or its representative to appear personally and make a time-limited 30-minute oral argument. The review panel shall recommend final action to the board.
- The board may affirm, modify, or reverse the recommendation of the review panel; or, in its discretion, refer the matter for further review and recommendation; or make its own decision based on the board's ultimate legal responsibility to grant appointment and clinical privileges.

### Final decision of the hospital board

Within 30 calendar days after receiving the review panel's recommendation, the board shall render a final decision in writing, including specific reasons for its action, and shall deliver copies to the affected individual and to the chairs of the credentials committee and the MEC, in person or by certified mail with return receipt requested.

### Right to one appeal only

No applicant or medical staff member shall be entitled as a matter of right to more than one hearing or appellate review on any single matter that may be the subject of an appeal. In the event that the board ultimately denies medical staff appointment or reappointment to an applicant, or revokes or terminates the medical staff appointment and/or clinical privileges of a current member, that individual may not apply within five years for medical staff appointment or for those clinical privileges at this hospital unless the board advises otherwise.

  

## Appeals to the Board

Most medical staff bylaws provide an opportunity for a practitioner to appeal an adverse determination by a fair hearing panel or a hearing officer. TJC requires hospitals to provide practitioners with an opportunity to appeal (MS.10.01.01), although there is no provision in HCQIA requiring an appellate review mechanism. The fair hearing and appeal process should delineate the following:

- The time frame in which the physician must submit the appeal request
- The grounds for which a physician may request an appeal
- The notification of the appeal's time, date, and place
- Whether the appeal can only be written or whether oral argument will also be allowed

## Reports to the NPDB

The medical staff bylaws should indicate when the hospital will submit reports to the NPDB regarding members of the medical staff. Writing NPDB reporting requirements into the bylaws has several advantages. First, it notifies medical staff members of the circumstances that call for an NPDB report. Second, regardless of any dispute over what the law may require, the hospital will have documentation showing that it acted properly if it filed a report with the NPDB consistent with the bylaws. When drafting this section, it is useful to peruse the language on reporting requirements in the NPDB guidebook and any applicable state statutes.

  

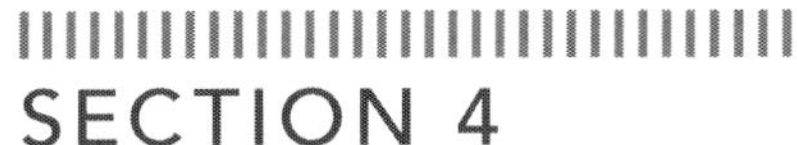

SECTION 4

# Credentialing and Privileging Procedures

One of the most important roles of a hospital's organized medical staff is to evaluate practitioners' credentials and make recommendations to the board regarding membership on the medical staff and/or the assignment of clinical privileges. Well-documented policies and procedures ensure compliance with accreditation standards and help practitioners provide high-quality healthcare. Credentialing policies should also help to:

- Establish clear lines of authority and accountability regarding credentialing
- Create an objective and documented credentialing process
- Provide an unambiguous direction for the medical staff services department (MSSD), department chairs, members of the credentials and executive committees, CEO, and board
- Promote high-quality, safe patient care by facilitating the appointment of well-qualified practitioners
- Minimize legal risk to the hospital and members of the medical staff

An organization's credentialing policies should address the following:

- The criteria that practitioners must meet to apply for medical staff membership and privileges.
- The information that the hospital requires of individuals applying for medical staff appointment.

- The levels of education, training, and experience—as well as the evidence of current competence—that the hospital requires practitioners to meet in order to be appointed to the medical staff or granted clinical privileges.

- The individuals who are responsible for collecting credentials information, verifying information supplied by the applicants, and ascertaining that all required information has been provided. The MSP performs verifications such as initial education, training, and experience; board certification (if required); National Practitioner Data Bank (NPDB) query; and Office of Inspector General (OIG) query.

- The individuals who are responsible for evaluating the information in a physician's application file and for making recommendations to the medical executive committee (MEC) regarding appointment and privileges.

- The duration of the application process.

The medical staff's credentialing policies should also address the reappointment process; specific privileging challenges, such as those posed by telemedicine, low-volume or no-volume practitioners, temporary privileges, emergency privileges, and disaster privileges; and special requests, such as leaves of absence.

In recent years, there has been substantial growth in the number of lawsuits filed against hospitals for alleged incidents of "negligent credentialing" after adverse events. Plaintiffs typically claim that the hospital failed to follow its own credentialing policies and procedures, and therefore appointed a physician who was not qualified to perform the procedure that led to the adverse outcome. Plaintiff's attorneys are also quick to point out incidents in which they believe an organization's credentialing policies fail to comply with accreditation standards. When policies are not written clearly or leave room for interpretation, or when they are too complex to follow easily, it is more likely that the hospital will deviate from expected practice.

  

An organization's credentialing procedures must be articulated with care. In this section, we highlight selected areas that should be covered in any credentialing discussion. In addition, sample bylaws or policy language is provided. This section follows the typical progression of the credentialing process: the application and data collection phase to verify information, the evaluation and recommendation of initial appointment, and the granting of privileges and reappointment.

## Establishing the Credentials Committee

Most medical staffs have a standing credentials committee, although some small staffs may use the MEC to directly manage credentialing tasks. It is not a requirement to have a credentials committee, although most medical staffs have one. If a credentials committee is established in the bylaws, a section of the credentialing procedures should clearly describe the committee's responsibilities, composition, and functions.

To ensure that the committee benefits from interested, experienced, and knowledgeable members, the members of the credentials committee should be able to serve significant tenures (e.g., three or more years). The medical staff should choose a chair who is skilled in credentialing, as opposed to a rotating medical staff officer who may have no background in credentialing and who cannot provide continuity of leadership to the committee. Credentialing is the area that subjects the medical staff to the greatest legal and regulatory scrutiny. It is also an area in which statutes and regulations are frequently revised. An experienced credentials committee chair can help the medical staff navigate these tempestuous waters.

It is common to see credentials committee chairs and members serve lengthier terms than other committees do, particularly because of the legal and regulatory standards that must be followed. Members should step on or off the credentials committee using a staggered rotation so that there are always experienced members on the committee. Medical staffs should consider rewarding leaders who choose to stay on the credentials committee for several successive terms, as it is a difficult job, and experience is strongly encouraged.

  

Some medical staffs try to ensure that the credentials committee is made up of practitioners from various specialties, and others require that every department is represented (which can make for an overly large committee). Some medical staffs compose these committees largely of experienced past medical staff officers. An increasing number of medical staffs assign the chair of the credentials committee a spot on the MEC to facilitate information between these two bodies. With these caveats in mind, there is no particular credentials committee composition that is ideal for all medical staffs.

The credentials committee has multiple responsibilities. First, it is responsible for developing and recommending policies and procedures for all credentialing and privileging activities, including the criteria for membership/privileges, which the board and medical staff approves. The credentials committee then uses these policies and criteria to judge applicants for membership/privileges and recommends approval or denial to the MEC. For Joint Commission–accredited organizations, the credentials committee is also involved in the initial focused professional practice evaluation (FPPE) assessment to ensure initial competency. Finally, according to most state laws, the credentials committee functions as a peer review committee.

Therefore, the information provided to and generated by the credentials committee must be protected. To enjoy those protections, the credentials committee must maintain confidentiality of the discussions and actions of the committee consistent with federal and state law.

## Putting the Competency Assessment to Work

All accrediting agencies require medical staffs to perform a global assessment of practitioner competence. Not only is this assessment required, ensuring the quality of care provided by those privileged through the medical staff is also the right thing to do.

In 2007, The Joint Commission (TJC) gave the field a structure by which to assess practitioner competence when it introduced what it called three new concepts in its revised credentialing and privileging standards. This structure has also been accepted by the American Osteopathic Association (AOA) for its graduate education programs. The first concept created a framework to measure practitioner competency and is modeled after the Accreditation Council for Graduate Medical Education and American Board of Medical Specialties (ABMS) joint initiative. This concept is known as the six areas of "general competencies," which are:

- Patient care
- Medical/clinical knowledge
- Practice-based learning and improvement
- Interpersonal and communication skills
- Professionalism
- Systems-based practice

Medical staffs should assess present and future practitioners using this framework or any other framework that assesses practitioner performance globally. If your hospital is Joint Commission–accredited, this framework does not have to be identical, but it must be comparable to the six general competencies.

The second concept that TJC introduced in 2007, ongoing professional practice evaluation (OPPE), is a process designed to continuously evaluate a practitioner's performance in the hope that the medical staff will identify and resolve potential problems as soon as possible. Although TJC does not use the term "peer review," OPPE is an attempt to improve the overall value of the peer review process.

The third concept, replaced the old "proctoring" with a more vigorous requirement called FPPE. There are two types of FPPE. One type evaluates the competence of all new practitioners to ensure initial competence. Initial FPPE is a defined period of FPPE that is required for any initially requested privilege, whether from a new applicant or from an existing privileged practitioner seeking a new privilege. The other type evaluates the performance of all practitioners who have been identified by an ongoing competency assessment to determine continued competence.

Medical staffs must establish FPPE criteria (akin to the old "focused review") to determine when to further evaluate practitioners if questions arise regarding practitioners' ability to provide safe, high-quality patient care during the course of OPPE.

Traditionally, the credentialing and privileging process has been a procedural, cyclical process in which practitioners are evaluated when they are initially granted privileges (FPPE) and every two years thereafter (OPPE).

If your organization is Joint Commission–accredited, it should enumerate all three of these concepts in the medical staff bylaws to ensure not only that the medical staff performs thorough peer review, but also that the medical staff has a solid defense if it is brought into litigation. If your organization is not Joint Commission–accredited, evaluating practitioner performance using a framework of performance criteria, initial review, ongoing review, and focused review (if necessary) are leading practices and comply with the competency assessment required by all regulators.

## SAMPLE BYLAWS LANGUAGE

### Focused professional practice evaluation

All initially requested privileges shall be subject to a period of focused professional practice evaluation (FPPE). The credentials committee, after receiving a recommendation from the department chair, and with the approval of the MEC, will define circumstances that require the clinical performance of each practitioner to be monitored and evaluated after he or she is initially granted privileges at the hospital. Such monitoring may use prospective, concurrent, or retrospective proctoring, including but not limited to the following:

- Chart review
- Tracking performance monitors/indicators
- External peer review
- Simulations
- Morbidity and mortality reviews
- Discussion with other healthcare workers involved in the care of patients

The credentials committee will also establish the duration for such FPPE, as well as triggers that indicate the need for performance monitoring.

  

## Qualifications for Membership and/or Privileges

Medical staff governing documents must articulate the standards that practitioners must meet to qualify for medical staff membership. In general, the list of qualifications will address the applicant's background, experience, ability to perform requested privileges, training, and demonstrated current competence; adherence to professional ethics; reputation; and any other factors appropriate to the effective operation of the hospital.

Each medical staff may set the standards for establishing the quality of its practitioners. Sometimes, the established criteria can cause dissent. For example, many medical staffs debate about whether to require members to be board certified. There is a growing trend nationally toward requiring all new medical staff members to achieve board certification either within a certain time after completing formal training (e.g., five years) or within a certain time period after joining the medical staff (e.g., five years). Practitioners who are already on the medical staff are generally grandfathered in when such a requirement is first implemented.

One confusing term that arises during these discussions is "board eligible." Some ABMS specialty boards have no time limits; others require applicants to apply for board certification within a specified time frame after they complete formal training and require them to complete their board certification within another time frame.

The AOA formally defines a "board eligible" physician as one who:

- Has completed an AOA-approved internship and residency
- Is a member in good standing of the AOA or the Canadian Osteopathic Association
- Has met the requirements of the applicable certifying board
- Has applied to and been accepted as a registrant by that board

The AOA has also imposed specific limits on the use of the term, requiring that candidates apply for certification within six years of finishing residency to be board eligible. The candidate's board eligible status ends six years after he or she first qualifies for board eligibility.

  

In general, when writing credentialing provisions, it is best to avoid the term "board eligible." If your medical staff allows some members to join who have completed residency but who have not fully completed all requirements for board certification, your credentialing policies should clearly state the expectations for completion.

The board certification issue has become more complex in recent years, as an increasing number of specialty boards have established recertification requirements. On January 1, 2010, the American Board of Pediatrics announced that newly issued certificates of board certification would not contain a specific end date. This means that a physician's board certification status will be linked to his or her status in the maintenance of certification (MOC) process, which can change over time depending on whether the physician is up to date in the MOC process. The AOA implemented a similar process called osteopathic continuous certification in 2013.

Although the majority of medical staffs require initial board certification within a specified time frame, it is much more variable whether they also require continued board recertification. There are multiple factors for the variation in board recertification requirements, including insurer mandates, subspecialization, robustness of the quality/peer review program, and cost. Your organization's credentialing policies should clearly state any requirements with regard to initial board certification/MOC.

Be aware of other terms that may cause confusion. For example, many credentialing policies require applicants to report any felony convictions, and those convictions may prevent a physician from being appointed to the medical staff. However, the definition of "felony" varies greatly from state to state. Often the individuals who draft credentialing policies are not aware of the scope of misbehavior to which their policies may be applied. Always check your state's laws when drafting medical staff bylaws to ensure that the bylaws comply with local laws and definitions of terms.

  

SAMPLE BYLAWS LANGUAGE

## Qualifications for membership and/or privileges

No practitioner shall be entitled to membership on the medical staff or to privileges merely by virtue of licensure, membership in any professional organization, or privileges at any other healthcare organization.

The following qualifications must be met by all practitioners who apply for medical staff appointment, reappointment, or clinical privileges:

- The applicant must demonstrate that he or she has successfully graduated from an approved school of medicine, osteopathy, [dentistry, podiatry, clinical psychology, optometry], or applicable recognized course of training in a clinical profession that is eligible to hold privileges.

- The applicant must have a current [unrestricted] state or federal license as a practitioner that is applicable to his or her profession and provides permission to practice within the state of [state name].

- The applicant must have a record that is free of current Medicare/Medicaid sanctions and not be on the Office of Inspector General's (OIG) list of excluded individuals/entities.

- The applicant must have a record that is free of felony convictions within the last three years, or occurrences that would raise questions of undesirable conduct that could injure the reputation of the medical staff or hospital. (***Author's Note:*** *The list of felonies and misdemeanors varies greatly from state to state. Therefore, each medical staff should customize the legal nomenclature to ensure its intent is achieved.*)

- The applicant must have fulfilled appropriate training requirements for various fields of practice along with any board certification requirements, if applicable.

- The applicant must possess a current, valid, [unrestricted] Drug Enforcement Administration number, if applicable.

- The applicant must have appropriate written and verbal communication skills.

SAMPLE BYLAWS LANGUAGE

## Qualifications for membership and/or privileges (cont.)

- The applicant must abstain from any participation in fee-splitting or other illegal payment, receipt, or remuneration with respect to referral or patient service opportunities.
- The applicant must possess a history of consistently acting in a professional, appropriate, and collegial manner with others in previous clinical and professional settings.
- The applicant must demonstrate his or her background, experience, training, current competence, knowledge, judgment, and ability to perform all privileges requested.
- The applicant must, on request, provide evidence of physical and mental health that does not impair, with reasonable accommodation, the fulfillment of his or her medical staff responsibilities and the specific privileges requested by and granted to the applicant.
- The applicant, if granted privileges, and who may have occasion to admit an inpatient must demonstrate his or her capability to provide continuous and timely care to the satisfaction of the MEC and the board.
- The applicant must demonstrate current clinical competence within the last 24 months in the area in which he or she seeks clinical privileges.
- The applicant must request privileges for a service the board has determined appropriate to provide at the hospital. The board must also see a need for this service under its medical staff development plan.
- The applicant must provide evidence of professional liability insurance appropriate to all privileges requested and of a type and in an amount established by the board after consulting with the MEC.

### Exceptions

- All practitioners who are current medical staff members and/or hold privileges as of [current date] and who have met prior qualifications for membership and/or privileges shall be exempt from board certification requirements.
- Only the board may create additional exceptions to the previous section after consulting with the MEC.

  

## *Application request procedure*

The credentialing documents should indicate how a practitioner who wants to join the medical staff may obtain an application. For example, a hospital may require an applicant to submit a written request or complete a pre-application. Many medical staffs have discontinued the use of pre-applications. Initially, medical staffs felt that if someone was not qualified, it was better to find out before the physician completed an application to avoid reporting that practitioner to NPDB when it had to deny him or her membership or privileges. However, regardless of whether a physician fills out a pre-application or a full application, if he or she is ineligible for membership and/or privileges, this is an ineligibility, not a denial, and therefore is not reportable to the NPDB. The added time and inconvenience of filling out and tracking both a pre-application and an application has caused many medical staffs to drop this process.

Yet, some staffs do not wish to go through the trouble of sending out and reviewing an application for someone who clearly does not meet the qualifications for staff membership. These hospitals may opt to send out a brief cover letter that lists the qualifications for membership with the application and informs applicants not to proceed with the application if

SAMPLE BYLAWS LANGUAGE

### Application request procedure

All requests for applications for appointment to the medical staff and requests for clinical privileges will be forwarded to the medical staff services department (MSSD). On receipt of the request, the MSSD will provide the applicant with an application package, which will include a complete set or overview of the medical staff bylaws or a reference to an electronic source for this information. This package will enumerate the eligibility requirements for medical staff membership, privileges, and performance expectations for individuals granted medical staff membership or privileges (if such expectations have been adopted by the medical staff).

If an applicant does not meet the board's membership or privileging criteria outlined in the application's cover letter, his or her application will not be processed and he or she will not be entitled to a fair hearing or any rights or due process provided under the medical staff bylaws.

  

they do not qualify. Other hospitals have an MSP who calls new applicants to ensure that it is appropriate to send out an application.

## Processing New Applications

The credentialing procedures should enumerate the information that the medical staff must obtain from practitioners during the application process. The language should clearly place on the applicant the burden of obtaining and providing the hospital with all the information requested in a timely manner.

A completed application includes the following:

- A completed, signed, and dated application form
- A completed privilege delineation form, if the practitioner is requesting privileges
- Copies of all requested documents and information necessary to confirm that the applicant meets the medical staff's criteria for membership and/or privileges and to establish current competency
- All applicable fees
- A copy of a current picture identification card issued by a state or federal agency (e.g., driver's license or passport) or current picture hospital identification card
- Receipt of all references (references shall come from peers knowledgeable about the applicant's experience, ability, and current competence to perform the requested privileges)
- Relevant practitioner-specific data as compared to aggregate data, when available
- Morbidity and mortality data from previous hospital, when available

An application should be deemed incomplete if any of the previous items are missing or if the need arises during the course of reviewing an application for additional or clarifiying information. As noted previously, the medical staff should not process an incomplete application, and not processing an application does not trigger a report to the NPDB or entitle the physician to a fair hearing. If, at any time during the credentialing process, it becomes apparent that an applicant does not meet all eligibility criteria for membership or privileges, the medical staff should terminate the credentialing process and take no further action.

The applicant is responsible for ensuring that the MSSD receives all required documents supporting the information he or she provided on the application. The applicant is also responsible for providing sufficient evidence that he or she meets the requirements for medical staff membership/the requested privileges.

If information is missing from the application, or the medical staff requires additional or clarifying information, the MSSD should send a letter requesting such information to the applicant. If the applicant does not return the requested information to the MSSD within a specified time frame, the medical staff should consider the application voluntarily withdrawn. This time frame varies among medical staffs.

## SAMPLE BYLAWS LANGUAGE

### Initial appointment procedure

On request, the medical staff services department will provide to prospective applicants an application package that includes the following:

- A blank application form with a cover letter outlining membership eligibility criteria
- A list of required supporting information
- A list of performance expectations for individuals granted medical staff membership and/or privileges (if such a list of expectations has been formally adopted by the medical staff)
- A description of responsibilities for medical staff members
- An overview of the delineation of privileges
- Privilege request form(s), including criteria for privileges
- A detailed list of requirements the physician must meet to complete the application, such as acknowledgment of receiving a copy of the bylaws and willingness to follow them and a statement attesting to the accuracy of the application

The applicant must complete and sign the application form. By signing this application:

- The applicant attests to the accuracy and completeness of all information on

SAMPLE BYLAWS LANGUAGE

## Initial appointment procedure (cont.)

the application and accompanying documents. The applicant agrees that any inaccuracy, omission, or misrepresentation, whether intentional or not, may be grounds for termination of the application process without the right to a fair hearing or appeal. If the inaccuracy, omission, or misstatement is discovered after an individual has been granted appointment and/or clinical privileges, the individual's appointment and privileges shall lapse effective as soon as he or she is notified, without the right to a fair hearing or appeal.

- The applicant consents to appear for any requested interviews in regard to his or her application.
- The applicant authorizes the hospital and medical staff representatives to consult with prior and current associates and others who may have information bearing on his or her professional competence, character, ability to perform the privileges requested, ethical qualifications, ability to work cooperatively with others, and other qualifications for membership and the clinical privileges that he or she requested.
- The applicant consents to hospital and medical staff representatives inspecting all records and documents that may be relevant to an evaluation of the following:
  - Professional qualifications and competence to carry out the clinical privileges requested
  - Physical, mental, and emotional health status that is relevant to safely perform requested privileges
  - Professional and ethical qualifications
  - Professional liability actions, including currently pending claims involving the applicant
  - Any other issue relevant to establishing the applicant's suitability for membership and/or privileges
- The applicant releases from liability, promises not to sue, and grants immunity to the hospital, its medical staff, and its representatives for acts performed and statements made in connection with the evaluation of the application and his or her credentials and qualifications to the fullest extent permitted by the law.

  

SAMPLE BYLAWS LANGUAGE

**Initial appointment procedure (cont.)**

- The applicant releases from liability and promises not to sue all individuals and organizations who provide information to the hospital or the medical staff. This information may include otherwise privileged or confidential information concerning his or her background, experience, competence, professional ethics, character, and physical and mental health to the extent relevant to fulfill requested privileges, emotional stability, utilization practice patterns, and other qualifications for staff appointment and clinical privileges.

- The applicant authorizes medical staff and administrative representatives to release credentialing and peer review information to other hospitals, medical associations, licensing boards, appropriate government bodies, and other healthcare entities concerned with this provider's performance and releases representatives of the hospital from liability for so doing.

- The applicant acknowledges that he or she has had access to the medical staff bylaws, including all rules, regulations, policies, and procedures of the medical staff, and agrees to abide by their provisions.

Notwithstanding these previous sections, if an individual institutes legal action and does not prevail, he or she shall reimburse the hospital and any member of the medical staff named in the action for all costs incurred defending such legal action, including reasonable attorney's fees.

On receipt of a completed application, the CEO, vice president of medical affairs (VPMA), credentials chair, or designee, in collaboration with the MSSD, must determine whether the applicant meets the requirements. In the event the applicant does not meet the requirements, the MSSD should notify the potential applicant that he or she is ineligible to apply for membership or privileges on the medical staff, the application will not be processed, and the applicant will not be eligible for a fair hearing. If the requirements are met, the MSSD should accept the application for further processing.

  

After receiving a completed application, the MSSD should verify the applicant's current licensure, education, relevant training, and current competence from the primary source, whenever feasible, or from a credentials verification organization. When it is not possible to obtain information from the primary source, the MSSD may use a reliable secondary source if it has documented its attempts to contact the primary source to no avail.

For example, if a school no longer exists or is in a foreign country where it is impossible to get information, the MSSD could receive verification from someone who did previously verify this information (i.e., the residency program, the licensing board) or a reference from a reliable colleague who knew the person in the foreign school. In addition, the MSSD should collect relevant additional information, which may include the following:

- Information from all prior and current liability insurance carriers concerning claims, suits, settlements, and judgments (if any) during the past 10 years.
- Documentation of the applicant's past clinical work experience.
- Licensure status in all states the practitioner has been or is currently licensed at the time the medical staff is in the process of granting membership or privileges. In addition, the MSSD should verify the practitioner's licensure with a primary source at the time of renewal or revision of clinical privileges, whenever a new privilege is requested, and at the time the applicant's license expires.
- Information from the AMA or AOA Physician Profile and the OIG's list of excluded individuals/entities.
- Information from professional training programs, including residency and fellowship programs.
- Information from the NPDB. In addition, the MSSD should query the NPDB at the time the applicant's privileges are renewed and whenever a new privilege(s) is requested.
- Other information regarding adverse credentialing and privileging decisions.
- One or more peer recommendations, as selected by the credentials committee, from practitioner(s) who have observed the applicant's clinical and professional performance and can evaluate the applicant's current medical/clinical knowledge, technical and

  

clinical skills, clinical judgment, interpersonal skills, communications skills, and professionalism, along with their physical, mental, and emotional ability to perform the requested privileges. (*Note:* Some medical staffs have confused the Joint Commission–mandated elements on a peer recommendation with the six general competencies. These are different and should be reviewed to ensure compliance.)

- Information from a criminal background check. (*Note:* This is not a regulatory requirement but is considered leading practice.)
- Information from any other sources relevant to the qualifications of the applicant to serve on the medical staff and/or hold privileges (e.g., licensing board, former coworkers, current medical staff members).
- Morbidity and mortality data and relevant practitioner-specific data as compared to aggregate data, when available.

Once the MSSD has appropriately collected and verified the previous items, the file must be reviewed. At this juncture, some credentials committees require the applicant to appear for an interview. When an interview is part of the medical staff credentialing procedures, it may be conducted by the appropriate department chair, the credentials committee, or any designee of the committee. The credentialing procedures regarding the initial appointment should outline the approach to applicant interviews (e.g., in person, over the phone, via video conferencing, etc.).

The role of the department chair in reviewing the application file, the actions of the credentials committee, and the MEC should also be outlined in the credentialing policy.

The Joint Commission requires that medical staff bylaws establish a specified time frame to complete applications; however, medical staffs are not required to assign timelines to the specific steps in the appointment process. Always use language that gives the organization appropriate latitude to adequately perform the necessary tasks.

  

SAMPLE BYLAWS LANGUAGE

### Processing applications

**Time periods for processing:** All individuals and groups acting on an application for staff appointment and/or clinical privileges must do so in a timely manner and in good faith. Except for a good cause, each application will be processed within 180 calendar days. These time periods are deemed guidelines and do not create any right for the practitioner to have an application processed within these time periods.

## Professional Practice Evaluation

In the past, medical staffs appointed new members for a provisional period, typically for six to 12 months, during which time they monitored the practitioner's performance. This provisional status/period need no longer exist because The Joint Commission's FPPE and OPPE regulations have replaced the monitoring provisions of the old provisional period with a more rigorous process.

Medical staffs must include some language in their bylaws regarding FPPE and OPPE if they are Joint Commission–accredited. The medical staff also needs to have continuing competency assessment, which The Joint Commission defines as OPPE, to identify professional practice trends that affect quality of care and patient safety. The medical staff should factor the information from this evaluation process into the decision to allow practitioners to maintain existing privileges, revise existing privileges, or revoke an existing privilege prior to or at the time of reappointment. OPPE should be undertaken as part of the medical staff's process to evaluate, measure, and improve practitioners' current clinical competency.

In addition, each practitioner may be subject to FPPE when issues affecting the provision of safe, high-quality patient care are identified during the OPPE process. Decisions to assign a period of performance monitoring or evaluation to further assess current competence must be based on the evaluation of an individual's current clinical competence, practice behavior, and ability to perform a specific privilege.

  

SAMPLE BYLAWS LANGUAGE

**Professional practice evaluation (cont.)**

All initially requested privileges shall be subject to a period of [focused professional practice evaluation. The credentials committee, after receiving a recommendation from the department chair and with the approval of the MEC, will define the circumstances that require monitoring and evaluation of the clinical performance of each practitioner following his or her initial grant of clinical privileges at the hospital. Such monitoring may involve prospective, concurrent, or retrospective proctoring, including but not limited to: chart review, the tracking of performance monitors/ indicators, external peer review, simulations, morbidity and mortality reviews, and discussion with other healthcare individuals involved in the care of each patient. The credentials committee will also establish the duration for such [focused professional practice evaluation] and triggers that indicate the need for performance monitoring.

The medical staff will also engage in [ongoing professional practice evaluation} to identify professional practice trends that affect quality of care and patient safety. Information from this evaluation process will be factored into the decision to maintain existing privileges, to revise existing privileges, or to revoke an existing privilege prior to or at the time of reappointment [ongoing professional practice evaluation] shall be undertaken as part of the medical staff's competency assessment process of evaluation, measurement, and improvement of a practitioner's performance. In addition, each practitioner may be subject to [focused professional practice evaluation] when issues affecting the provision of safe, high-quality patient care are identified through the [ongoing professional practice evaluation] process. Decisions to assign a period of performance monitoring or evaluation to further assess current competence must be based on the evaluation of an individual's current clinical competence, practice behavior, and ability to perform a specific privilege.

## Processing Reappointments

Historically, many medical staffs reappointed staff members with little thought. If the member's department chair was not aware of significant problems, the practitioner's reappointment sailed through committee review. Today, medical staffs are expected to rigorously reappraise the appropriateness of each practitioner's ongoing membership and assignment of privileges. Typically, the credentials policy requires practitioners to submit a reappointment application that updates the information collected in the original application. At the same time, the physician must reapply for all the privileges he or she will want. These policies usually enable the MSSD and the credentials committee to collect additional information so that a robust reappraisal can occur.

During the reappointment process, the MSSD should collect and verify the following information:

- Information from the ongoing competency assessment process, including clinical activity in the institution and performance data on all the competency categories used to evaluate practitioners
- Performance and conduct in the hospital and other healthcare organizations in which the practitioner has provided clinical care since the last reappointment
- Documentation of any required hours of continuing medical education activity
- Service on medical staff, department, and hospital committees
- Timely and accurate completion of medical records
- Compliance with all applicable bylaws, policies, rules, regulations, and procedures of the hospital and medical staff
- Significant gaps in employment or practice since the previous appointment or reappointment
- Verification of current licensure
- NPDB query
- Malpractice history for the past two years, which the MSSD primary source verifies with the practitioner's malpractice carrier(s)

  

When sufficient peer review data are not available to evaluate a practitioner's competence, the MSSD should obtain one or more peer recommendations (as selected by the credentials committee) from practitioners who have observed the applicant's clinical and professional performance and can evaluate the applicant's current medical/clinical knowledge, technical and clinical skills, clinical judgment, interpersonal skills, communication skills. and professionalism, as well as their physical, mental, and emotional ability to perform the requested privileges.

## Clinical Privileges for Practitioners Who Are Not Members of the Medical Staff

Deciding who should be granted clinical privileges is one of the most important quality-control mechanisms executed by the medical staff. Remember, privileges are different and distinct from membership. Although membership establishes a practitioner's social hierarchy in the organization (whether the practitioner may vote, hold office, serve on committees, etc.), privileges grant the practitioner a "work ticket."

Privileges can be granted to individuals who are not members of the medical staff, such as locum tenens physicians who are granted privileges to treat patients for a specified period but are not granted medical staff membership. With the advent of telemedicine/teleradiology, it seems only practical to grant these practitioners privileges, yet not include them as members of the medical staff because they may never set foot in the hospital. Other advanced practice professionals, such as physician's assistants and advanced practice registered nurses, are granted privileges through the medical staff process, yet frequently these individuals are not members of the medical staff. The credentialing and privileging process, as well as the fair hearing and appeal process for non-physician practitioners, is dealt with in Section 5 of this book.

## Requests for New Privileges

Requests for clinical privileges should be considered only when accompanied by evidence of the physician's education, training, experience, and demonstrated current competence as specified by the hospital in its board-approved criteria for clinical privileges.

When a physician who is already a member of your medical staff or a new physician requests privileges for a new technology, those new privilege requests may affect only one specialty, so it is up to that specialty to recommend privileging criteria to the credentialing committee. However, sometimes the new privilege requests affect more than one specialty. In these circumstances, the medical staff should develop new cross-specialty criteria.

To approve criteria for a new procedure, two processes must occur. First, the hospital must consider two questions:

1. Is the new privilege within the hospital's mission and values, as well as its strategic, operating, capital, information, and staffing plans?

2. Did the board determine that the privilege will benefit patients, the community, and the hospital?

The medical staff must also answer some questions as it evaluates whether a new privilege should be allowed:

- Is the new privilege better than existing privileges?

- Does it offer better quality?

- Does it offer equivalent quality but is less invasive, less costly, or leads to increased patient satisfaction?

- Is the new privilege under an existing exclusive contract?

  

- What should be criteria for eligibility to obtain the new privilege?
- Does the development of eligibility criteria affect more than one specialty?

During the process of determining privileging criteria, the following steps are leading practice:

- In the event a physician submits a request for a privilege for a new technology, a procedure new to the hospital, or an existing procedure used in a significantly different manner, or the request involves a cross-specialty privilege for which no criteria have been established, the MEC will table the request for a reasonable period, usually not to exceed 60 calendar days. During this time the MEC will:
  - Review the community, patient, and hospital need for the privilege and reach an agreement with management and the board that the privilege is approved to be exercised at the hospital
  - Review the efficacy and clinical viability of the requested privilege with members of the credentials committee and confirm that the appropriate regulatory agencies (FDA, OSHA, etc.) approve the use of the privilege in the setting-specific area of the hospital
  - Meet with management to ensure that the new privilege is consistent with the hospital's mission and values, as well as its strategic, operating, capital, information, and staffing plans
  - Work with management to ensure that all exclusive contract issues, if applicable, are resolved in such a way as to allow the new or cross-specialty privileges in question to be provided without violating the existing contract
  - Formulate the necessary criteria and recommend them to the board on recommendation from the credentials committee and the appropriate department, specialty, or subject matter experts as determined by the credentials committee

  

- For the development of criteria, the MSP (or designee) will compile information relevant to the privileges requested, which may include, but need not be limited to the following:
  - Position and opinion papers from specialty organizations
  - White papers from organizations such as HCPro's Credentialing Resource Center and other sources, as available
  - Position and opinion statements from interested individuals or groups
  - Documentation from other hospitals in the region, as appropriate
- Criteria to be established for the privilege(s) in question include education, training, board status, certification (if applicable), experience, and evidence of current competence. Initial competency assessment (such as FPPE) requirements, if any, will be addressed, including who may serve as a proctor and how many proctored cases will be required. Hospital-related issues such as exclusive contracts, equipment, clinical support staff, and management will be referred to the appropriate hospital administrator and/or department/clinical service director.
- If the privileges requested overlap two or more specialty disciplines, the credentials chair will appoint an ad hoc committee to recommend criteria for the privilege(s) in question. This committee will consist of one or two members from each involved discipline. The chair of the ad hoc committee should be a member of the credentials committee who has no vested interest in the issue.
- The credentials committee should review the criteria for recommendation to the MEC.
- The MEC should review the criteria for recommendation to the board.
- The board should review and approve, if appropriate, the criteria for the new privilege.

  

- Once objective criteria have been established, the original request from the practitioner will be processed as described herein.

- The credentials committee will evaluate requests for clinical privileges on the basis of the practitioner's prior and continuing education and training; experience and utilization practice patterns; current ability to perform the privileges requested; and demonstrated current competence, ability, and judgment. The credentials committee may also consider additional factors when recommending privileges, such as patient care needs, the hospital's ability to support the type of privileges being requested, and the availability of qualified coverage in the applicant's absence. The basis for determining privileges in connection with periodic reappointment or a requested change in privileges must include documented clinical performance and results of the staff's performance improvement program activities. The credentials committee should also base privileges recommendations on pertinent information from other sources, such as peers and/or faculty from other institutions and healthcare settings where the practitioner exercises clinical privileges.

## Special Conditions for Residents or Fellows in Training

An organization's credentialing and privileging policies should address various special circumstances. If a hospital provides medical education, it may be necessary to address the roles of residents and fellows. Residents and fellows in training do not normally hold membership on the medical staff and are not normally granted specific clinical privileges. Rather, they are permitted to function clinically only in accordance with the written training protocols developed by the VPMA, chief education officer, a professional graduate education committee, or the medical director in conjunction with the residency training program.

The protocols should delineate the roles, responsibilities, and patient care activities of residents and fellows, including which types of residents may write patient care orders, under what circumstances they may do so, and what entries a supervising physician must cosign. The protocol should also describe the mechanisms through which resident directors and supervisors make decisions about a resident's progressive involvement and independence when delivering patient care and how these decisions will be communicated to appropriate medical staff and hospital leaders.

The residency program director or graduate medical education committee must communicate periodically with the MEC and the board about the performance of its residents, patient safety issues, and quality of patient care. It must also work with the MEC to ensure that all supervising physicians possess clinical privileges commensurate with their supervising activities.

## Special Conditions for Moonlighting Residents and Fellows

Residents and fellows who are working in the hospital in a capacity outside their training programs must be credentialed using the medical staff process. If they are still in their training period, they do not qualify for medical staff membership because they have not completed their training. However, they can be privileged in the same fashion as others who do not qualify for medical staff membership. The medical staff should define what level of training is adequate for privileging and process them like all other candidates.

Usually residents and fellows in training who moonlight in the organization are either not eligible for medical staff membership (residents) or uninterested in medical staff membership (fellows); they are typically only interested in privileges that allow them to moonlight. They are not assigned to a medical staff category because they are not members. They still retain the full fair hearing and appeal rights as full members do because they are privileged through the medical staff and qualify for the due process rights as other physicians do, furnished by the Health Care Quality Improvement Act of 1986.

## Temporary Privileges

Another example of special circumstances regarding privileges involves granting temporary privileges. Language regarding temporary privileges should be crafted in accordance with current regulatory standards. Notably, in recent years, many hospitals have been found to be noncompliant on this issue when they are visited by accreditation surveyors. Temporary privileges are intended to fulfill the needs of patients or providers in specific circumstances. Temporary privileges should not be used routinely or as an expected convenience measure. The rule of thumb is to never grant temporary privileges to someone you would not feel comfortable granting regular privileges to.

When granting temporary privileges, the CEO (or designee) acts on behalf of the board, usually based on the recommendation of the president of the medical staff (or designee). For TJC–accredited hospitals, temporary privileges may be granted in only two circumstances:

- To fulfill an important patient care, treatment, or service need
- When an initial applicant with a complete application that raises no concerns is awaiting review and approval of the MEC and the board

The hospital may grant temporary privileges on a case-by-case basis when an important patient care, treatment, or service need exists that mandates an immediate authorization to practice. The definition of an important patient care, treatment, or service need varies among medical staffs. The time a practitioner can practice under temporary privileges cannot exceed 120 calendar days. When granting temporary privileges, the organized medical staff needs only to verify current licensure and current competence (although most MSSDs do as much verification as time allows).

The second circumstance is less urgent. If a physician has a clean application and is simply waiting for review and recommendation from the MEC and approval from the board, the CEO, following a recommendation from the medical staff president, may grant the physician temporary privileges for up to 120 calendar days. The information needed to grant temporary privileges in this circumstance differs from the baseline verifications needed to grant temporary privileges for an important patient care need. To receive temporary privileges under these circumstances, the applicant must have submitted a complete application that was verified and determined to be a "clean" file by the department chair and credentials committee. It is recommended that the policy define a "clean" file.

  

It is noted that TJC allows temporary privileges for up to 120 days. Det Norske Veritas (DNV) allows an initial grant, by the CEO, of temporary privileges of 30 days. DNV then allows two additional 30-day grants of temporary privileges, but these must be granted by the board. The total amount of time allowed for temporary privileges by DNV is 90 days. It is noted that HFAP has just recently changed from 90 days to 120 days for the extent of temporary privileges.

## Expedited Credentialing

Although TJC allows the two types of temporary privileges noted previously, it prefers that medical staffs use the expedited credentialing process instead of temporary privileges for practitioners with clean applications awaiting approval of the MEC and board. Expedited credentialing is an expedited board process; the remainder of the credentialing process still must occur. If, during the normal privileging process, a department chair signs off on an applicant's privileges, this action must still occur during the expedited credentialing process. If your medical staff has a credentials committee, it must get approval from the credentials committee. Medical staffs can write into the bylaws that the credentials chair can approve clean applications on behalf of the entire committee. The MEC must also approve the expedited credentialing application; however, it can delegate this responsibility to a limited number of committee members who review these clean applications on behalf of the entire committee (again, if written in the bylaws to do so). Finally, expedited credentialing applications can go to a subcommittee of the board made up of at least two members that can act on behalf of the whole board.

These other processes must be written in the bylaws to occur. If they are, once an application is complete and verified, the remainder of the process can occur as quickly as one or two days and should occur on an as needed basis rather than on a schedule.

Many medical staffs separate applications into two categories to allow for expedited credentialing of uncomplicated applicants. A "clean" or "category 1" application is one that contains no red flags. The applicant submitting such an application is eligible for expedited approval if this is permitted under the medical staff's credentialing procedures.

If your facility is Joint Commission–accredited (HFAP and DNV do not have expedited credentialing requirements), there are two conditions that exclude an individual from expedited credentialing: an incomplete application or an adverse final recommendation from the MEC. TJC states that the following should be evaluated on a case-by-case basis and usually result in ineligibility for the expedited credentialing process:

- A current challenge or a previously successful challenge to licensure or registration
- Involuntary termination of medical staff membership at another hospital
- An involuntary limitation, reduction, denial, or loss of clinical privileges
- An unusual pattern of, or an excessive number of, professional liability actions resulting in a final judgment against the applicant

A "category 2" application is either incomplete; raises red flags regarding the practitioner's clinical competence, professionalism, or conduct; or has not been brought to the medical staff's attention because the practitioner did not request an expedited process. The department chair, the full credentials committee, the full MEC, and the board all review and act on applications that fall into category 2.

## Emergency and Disaster Privileges

In addition to temporary privileges, the medical staff credentials policies should address emergency and disaster privileges. Frequently, emergency and disaster privileges are confused. Emergency privileges are those privileges that the medical staff has granted to already existing members to do whatever is necessary (within the scope of each practitioner's license) to save the life, limb, or organ of a patient. Typically, the practitioner is required to ask an appropriately privileged colleague to consult on or become involved with a case at the earliest feasible time.

Disaster privileges are those privileges that the medical staff grants to individuals outside its existing privileged providers to work during a declared emergency. Disaster privileges enable a hospital to quickly take advantage of volunteer assistance when it is faced with a crisis that overwhelms its internal abilities to provide professional care. The Joint Commission has issued standards by which such disaster privileges can be deployed, and bylaws language should mirror these standards. Specifically, you will need to delineate the following:

- What identification the medical staff requires before granting a physician disaster privileges
- What badging is needed to identify the practitioner while he or she practices in the facility
- The time frame in which the MSSD should complete verifications
- How the performance of these outside practitioners will be monitored in the facility

## SAMPLE BYLAWS LANGUAGE

### Disaster privileges

If the institution's disaster plan has been activated, and the organization is unable to meet immediate patient needs, the CEO and other individuals as identified in the institution's disaster plan with similar authority may, on a case-by-case basis, grant disaster privileges to selected licensed independent practitioners (LIP). The granting of privileges must be consistent with medical licensing and other relevant state statutes. The LIPs must present a valid government-issued photo identification issued by a state or federal agency (e.g., driver's license or passport) and at least one of the following:

- A current picture hospital ID card that clearly identifies professional designation
- A current license to practice
- Primary source verification of the license
- Identification indicating that the individual is a member of a Disaster Medical Assistance Team, Medical Reserve Corps, Emergency System for Advance Registration of Volunteer Health Professionals or other recognized state or federal organizations or groups

  

SAMPLE BYLAWS LANGUAGE

### Disaster privileges (cont.)

- Identification indicating that the individual has been granted authority to render patient care, treatment, and services in disaster circumstances (such authority having been granted by a federal, state, or municipal entity)
- Identification by a current hospital or medical staff member(s) who possesses personal knowledge regarding the volunteer's ability to act as a LIP during a disaster

The medical staff oversees the professional performance of volunteer practitioners who have been granted disaster privileges by direct observation, mentoring, or clinical record review.

The organization makes a decision (based on information obtained regarding the professional practice of the volunteer) within 72 hours whether disaster recovery privileges should be continued.

Primary source verification of licensure begins as soon as the immediate situation is under control, and is completed within 72 hours from the time the volunteer practitioner presents to the organization.

Once the immediate situation has passed and such determination has been made consistent with the institution's disaster plan, the practitioner's disaster privileges will terminate immediately.

Any individual identified in the institution's disaster plan with the authority to grant disaster privileges shall also have the authority to terminate disaster privileges. Such authority may be exercised in the sole discretion of the hospital and will not give rise to a right to a fair hearing or an appeal.

## Special Conditions for the Aging Practitioner

More practitioners are working well into their golden years. In many cases, they are still excellent practitioners, but some may have difficulty keeping up with the volume of medical information and changes in practice or experience age-related physical concerns. This is especially true if they have been out of training.

Many medical staffs have chosen to proactively perform a focused review of all practitioners who reach a certain number of years post training, to ensure that these practitioners continue to deliver good patient care and that the medical staff reviews all practitioners fairly. In some medical staffs, these same practitioners are required to undergo evaluation of their clinical performance to assess their capacity to perform their requested privileges. Such an evaluation is required even in the absence of any previous performance concerns. The scope and duration of the evaluation is determined by the MEC and the credentials committee, and their decision is based on the department chair's recommendation.

In addition to the competency evaluation, practitioners may be required to complete an annual examination that addresses their physical and mental capacity to perform the privileges they have requested. The physical and mental exams should be conducted by a physician who is deemed acceptable to the credentials committee and/or MEC. The physical exam is a "fitness to work" evaluation and must indicate that the practitioner has no physical or mental problems that may interfere with the safe and effective provision of care permitted under the privileges granted.

## Telemedicine Privileges

Practitioners who provide readings of images, tracings, or specimens through a telemedicine mechanism must be credentialed through the regular medical staff process. The Centers for Medicare & Medicaid Services allows telemedicine providers to be credentialed in three different ways:

  

1. Credential the telemedicine provider with full verification by the medical staff

2. Credential the telemedicine provider using static information (education, training, work history) from the telemedicine entity, supplement with current verifications, and continue through the medical staff process

3. Credential the telemedicine provider by accepting the credentialing decision of the telemedicine entity (when certain other provisions are met)

Across the country, most medical staffs are utilizing the second option since it offers some efficiency in the collection of the static information but it allows the medical staff to make its own independent decision on whether to privilege the telemedicine provider.

## Leaves of Absence

Requests for leaves of absence have become more common in recent years, and it is important for medical staffs to have clear policies regarding their use. A member of the medical staff may request a leave of absence for personal reasons, such as the birth of a child, illness of a family member, participation in an extended mission project overseas, pursuit of additional education, or fulfillment of required military service. A leave of absence may also be required if the medical staff member must participate in an impaired practitioner program.

Some medical staffs ask practitioners to take a leave of absence so that they can participate in a remedial education program when the medical staff has raised concerns about the quality of their performance. In general, a leave of absence is not reportable to the NPDB and, in many states, it is also not reportable to the board of medicine. Your bylaws or associated manuals should specify how practitioners may request a leave of absence and who may authorize it. The acceptable duration for the leave should be specified in the bylaws, as well.

If a practitioner fails to request reinstatement to the medical staff during his or her leave of absence, the medical staff typically treats the situation as an automatic resignation. The bylaws language should make clear that the termination of a leave of absence is at the discretion of the board. The board may require evidence of activities that took place during the leave. For example, if the practitioner was participating in a rehabilitation program, it will ask the program to provide documentation showing the dates the physician participated. The board may place appropriate conditions on practitioners if they are to resume their appointment.

## SAMPLE BYLAWS LANGUAGE

### Leaves of absence

**Leave request:** A leave of absence must be requested for any absence from the medical staff and/or patient care responsibilities longer than 30 days if such absence is related to the individual's physical or mental health or to his or her ability to care for patients safely and competently. A practitioner who wishes to obtain a voluntary leave of absence must provide written notice to the president of the medical staff stating the reasons for the leave and approximate duration of the leave, which may not exceed one year, except for military service or express permission from the board. Requests for leaves must be forwarded with a recommendation from the MEC and affirmed by the board. While on leave of absence, the practitioner may not exercise clinical privileges and has no obligation to fulfill medical staff responsibilities. In the event that a practitioner has not demonstrated good cause for a leave of absence, or when a request for an extension is not granted, the determination shall be final, and the practitioner will have no recourse to a hearing and appeal.

**Termination of leave:** At least 30 calendar days prior to the termination of the leave, or at any earlier time, the practitioner may request to be reinstated by sending a written notice to the president of the medical staff. The practitioner must submit a written summary of relevant activities during the leave if the MEC or board so requests. A practitioner returning from a leave of absence for health reasons must provide a report from his or her physician that answers any questions that the MEC or board may have as part of considering the request for reinstatement. The MEC makes a recommendation to the board concerning reinstatement, and the applicable privileging procedures are followed. If the practitioner's current grant of membership and/or privileges is due to expire during the leave of absence, the practitioner must apply for reappointment, or his or her appointment and/or clinical privileges shall lapse at the end of the appointment period.

  

## Practitioners Providing Contracted Services

Some practitioners who exercise privileges at a hospital do so under contractual arrangements. In some cases, the contracts stipulate limitations on the privileges that the practitioner may hold. Sometimes, contracts express privileging criteria that are more rigorous than those generally adopted by the medical staff. However, such contracts should never allow criteria that are less rigorous than those that the medical staff has already adopted.

When a hospital grants exclusive contracts, the privileges of other members of the medical staff may be affected. The medical staff credentialing procedures should ensure that all parties have proper notice regarding the effect that contracts will have on privileges.

Whenever hospital policy specifies that certain hospital facilities or services may be provided on an exclusive basis in accordance with contracts or letters of agreement between the hospital and qualified practitioners, then other practitioners must, except in an emergency or life-threatening situation, adhere to the exclusivity policy when arranging for or providing care. The MSSD should not accept or process applications for initial appointment or for clinical privileges related to the hospital services covered by exclusive agreements unless a physician submits an application in accordance with the existing contract or agreement with the hospital. Practitioners who have previously been granted privileges that now become covered by an exclusive contract will not be able to exercise those privileges unless they become a party to the contract.

A practitioner who is or will be providing specified professional services pursuant to a contract or a letter of agreement with the hospital must meet the same qualifications, have his or her application processed in the same manner, and fulfill all the obligations of his or her appointment category as any other applicant or staff appointee.

The effect of expiration or other termination of a contract on a practitioner's staff appointment and clinical privileges will be governed solely by the terms of the practitioner's contract with the hospital. If the contract or the employment agreement is silent on the matter, then contract expiration or other termination alone will not affect the practitioner's staff appointment status or clinical privileges. The physician will continue to have privileges at the hospital despite the terminated contract.

  

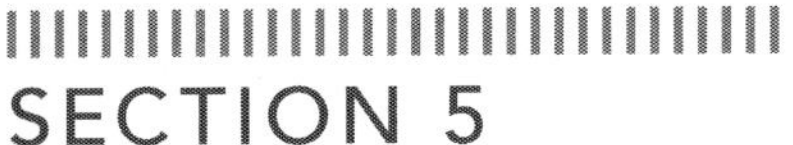

SECTION 5

# Allied Health Professionals

Many organizations ask how and where allied health professionals (AHP) fit in to the medical staff bylaws. The term AHP means different things to different organizations, and this type of practitioner goes by a variety of names. In general, AHPs are usually not members of the medical staff.

There are two distinct groups of AHPs. One group consists of practitioners who must be granted privileges through the medical staff process in accordance with The Joint Commission's (TJC) and Healthcare Facilities Accreditation Program's standards, and can be called advanced practice professionals (APP). An APP is an individual, other than a licensed physician, (or dentist or podiatrist if members of the medical staff) who provides direct patient care services in the hospital under a defined degree of supervision by a physician medical staff member with clinical privileges. These individuals are clinical psychologists, physician's assistants, advanced practice registered nurses (and dentists and podiatrists if not members of the medical staff). APPs exercise judgment within their specific areas of documented professional competence and consistent with the applicable State Practice Act.

APPs are designated by the board to be credentialed and privileged through the medical staff and are granted clinical privileges as defined in the medical staff bylaws. The board periodically reevaluates the categories of APPs eligible for clinical privileges. APPs may be employed by or have contracts with the hospital, or they may be employed, contracted, or sponsored by members of the medical staff. Even though these practitioners are granted privileges, these individuals are usually not medical staff members and therefore need not be assigned to any medical staff category.

The second group of AHPs consists of individuals that the hospital does not need to privilege through the medical staff but who provide services that are consistent with a scope of care approved by the medical staff and the board. These individuals should perhaps be called clinical assistants (CA). CAs must be qualified by academic education and clinical experience, or other training as specified in the approved scope of practice or job description, to provide patient care services in a clinical or supportive role. CAs are typically not credentialed and privileged through the medical staff services department. Rather, their services are approved by the hospital's human resources department.

CAs provide services only under the supervision of a member of the medical staff and provide only those clinical services that are consistent with a written scope of practice or job description approved by the board. The individuals who may be eligible include surgical assistants/technicians, registered nurse first assistants (RNFA), private duty scrub technicians, perfusionists, and occupational and physical therapists.

It is noted that the Centers for Medicare & Medicaid Services requires surgical technicians and RNFAs who perform a medical level of care (such as manipulate tissue, provide hemostatis, perform litigation, or suture) must be privileged through the medical staff process.

## SAMPLE BYLAWS LANGUAGE

### Credentialing advanced practice professionals

**Basic qualifications of an advanced practice professional (APP):** An APP shall not be employed, granted authority to exercise privileges, or given a credentialing application unless and until the board has authorized and approved the provision of such services. The following are APP categories consistent with this policy:

- Psychologists
- Physician's assistants
- Advanced practice registered nurses
  - Nurse-midwives

  

SAMPLE BYLAWS LANGUAGE

## Credentialing advanced practice professionals (cont.)

- Nurse practitioners
- Nurse anesthetists
- Clinical nurse specialists

**Demonstration of qualifications:** At all times, the APP is responsible for demonstrating the following qualifications:

- Continued employment by the hospital or an employment, contract, or sponsorship with a member of the medical staff organization
- Requisite professional education and training, licensure and/or certification, and registration, as applicable
- Demonstrated clinical ability and judgment
- Relevant experience demonstrated by clinical activity
- Current competence to practice his or her profession and perform all requested clinical privileges
- Freedom from any significant physical, emotional, or behavioral impairment (including the use of drugs or alcohol) that prevents the APP from meeting the other qualifications for APP status and the requested privileges
- Acceptable professional claims history and continuous professional liability coverage in prescribed amounts
- Adherence to the lawful ethics of the APP profession
- The ability to work cooperatively with others in the organization and with

SAMPLE BYLAWS LANGUAGE

## Credentialing advance practice professionals (cont.)

healthcare professionals in a consistently cordial and productive manner

**Professional liability insurance requirements:** APPs who are employed by the hospital are covered for professional liability for services provided as an employee under insurance policies of the applicable organization(s). APPs who are employed, contracted, or sponsored by members of the medical staff must be covered by the practitioner's employer and specifically named in the professional liability policy and must meet organizational requirements for coverage. APPs must demonstrate independent professional liability insurance in the amount required by the medical staff and governing body.

**Basic responsibilities:** Each APP shall:

- Provide patients with quality care at the generally recognized professional level of quality and efficiency in the community to the extent authorized by his or her license, certification, or other legal credentials
- Abide by all applicable state and federal laws that regulate healthcare providers, as well as the hospital's rules and regulations and all other lawful standards, policies, and rules
- Perform functions assigned by the medical executive committee (MEC), including, but not limited to, quality improvement, peer and professional review, patient care monitoring, utilization review, case management, and other responsibilities
- Participate in committee activities as requested by the MEC
- Submit to physical and/or mental examination(s) or provide verification of health status as may be required to verify the APP's ability to fully meet his or her

  

SAMPLE BYLAWS LANGUAGE

## Credentialing advance practice professionals (cont.)

responsibilities and/or perform the requested privileges

- Report immediately any action taken that affects licensure, certification, registration, or Drug Enforcement Administration (DEA) registration to medical staff services, including, but not limited to, probation, restriction, suspension, termination, and voluntary or involuntary relinquishment of privileges
- Use hospital resources appropriately
- Treat all individuals at or associated with the hospital courteously, respectfully, and with dignity at all times
- Comply with medical staff and hospital bylaws, policies, procedures, rules, regulations, and requirements that relate to the provision of services rendered by APPs at the hospital
- Write orders only as permitted by his or her licensure or certification
- Document inpatient medical records completely and in a timely fashion, to the extent authorized
- Seek consultation, supervision, and direction whenever appropriate or necessary
- Abide by the ethical principles of his or her profession
- Observe and promote the confidentiality of patient-identifiable information at all times

**Relationship to medical staff:** APPs are not members of the medical staff and do not have voting privileges at medical staff meetings. APPs may attend medical staff

SAMPLE BYLAWS LANGUAGE

## Credentialing advance practice professionals (cont.)

meetings only when appointed to a committee or department or requested to attend by an authorized representative of the medical staff organization, such as an officer, department chair, or committee chair.

**Supervision procedures:** APPs must be assigned to a medical staff member who serves as a supervisor/collaborator/sponsor and is deemed acceptable by the medical staff. The supervisor/collaborator/sponsor must be a member of the active medical staff in good standing. The supervisor/collaborator/sponsor must sign the privileges of the APP he or she supervises. In doing so, he or she accepts responsibility for appropriate supervision of the services provided by each APP under his or her supervision and agrees that the APP will not exceed the scope of practice defined by law and within the APP's supervising/collaborating/sponsoring agreement. The supervisor/collaborator/sponsor must agree to participate as requested in the evaluation of the APP's competence (i.e., during and at the conclusion of the initial [focused professional practice evaluation], at the time of reappointment, and at intervals between reappointment, as necessary). A copy of the supervising/collaborating/sponsoring agreement will be submitted, and the APP's application will be signed by both parties.

**Reappointment:** The medical staff services department follows the reappointment procedures for APPs as defined in the hospital's credentialing policies and procedures. Following this policy includes gathering data for all credentialed medical staff members and APPs as applicable to the services provided and the data available.

  

## Procedures for Evaluating Performance

The medical staff should evaluate the performance of all APPs as part of its routine performance improvement processes. APPs' performance should be consistent with the medical staff policies and procedures regarding competency assessment (focused and ongoing professional practice evaluation, if your hospital is Joint Commission–accredited). Any concerns regarding the quality or appropriateness of care provided by an APP identified during this review process should be brought to the attention of the appropriate medical staff review committee.

If an individual has concerns regarding a physician's supervision of an APP, he or she should report those concerns to the appropriate medical staff department or review committee. In addition, the hospital likely evaluates the quality of care provided by the APPs that it employs on an ongoing basis through its employment performance evaluation process.

## Automatic Relinquishment of Privileges

The board should not grant APPs the right to dispute automatic relinquishment of privileges. Automatic relinquishment would occur if the license or other legal credential of the APP expired or was revoked, or if the APP was excluded from Medicare/Medicaid, etc. Automatic termination would occur if the APP failed to meet his or her eligibility criteria.

The board should terminate an APP's privileges and status immediately, without right to a fair hearing, in the event that the APP's employment with the hospital is terminated for any reason, or if the APP's employment, contract, or sponsorship with a member of the medical staff organization is terminated for any reason.

## Corrective Action

Whenever the activities or professional conduct of an APP adversely affects, or is likely to adversely affect, patient safety or the delivery of quality patient care, or if the APP's professional conduct is disruptive to the organization's operations, the matter should be referred to the credentials committee or medical executive committee for consideration of corrective action. The credentials committee should review the matter or designate an ad hoc or existing peer review body to evaluate the matter.

The credentials committee may use external third parties to conduct all or part of the investigation or to provide information to the investigating body. The investigation may include an interview with the APP involved, his or her supervising/collaborating/sponsoring medical staff member, and/or other individuals or groups who can potentially provide valuable information regarding the APP's performance.

## Fair Hearing and Appeal Process

The hospital/medical staff should allow APPs the right to dispute any action that revokes, suspends, terminates, restricts, or reduces the clinical privileges that they have been given permission to provide at the hospital, unless the action revokes, suspends, terminates, restricts, or reduces the clinical privileges of an entire classification of APPs rather than being focused on an individual.

Organizations must consider the section of the bylaws that relates to hearing and appeals for APPs carefully.For example, TJC's medical staff standards permit a different right of hearing and appeal for individuals who are members of the medical staff versus those who are not members but are privileged by the medical staff. However, medical staffs must give practitioners the right to a hearing and appeal. Although some medical staff organizations provide the same right of hearing and appeal to APPs, others choose to provide a less extensive process. The following are factors to consider when making this determination:

- Will the outcome be reported to the National Practitioner Data Bank? If the answer is yes, the hearing must meet the requirements stated in the Health Care Quality Improvement Act of 1986. Most likely, the APP would receive the same hearing and appeal rights as members of the medical staff.

  

- Are there state-specific laws or regulations affecting the right to a hearing and appeal?

Carefully weigh and discuss these factors with the hospital's legal counsel to determine the best course for the organization.

## SAMPLE BYLAWS LANGUAGE

### Fair hearing and appeal process for APPs

Advanced practice professionals [are/are not] entitled to the hearing and appeals procedures set forth in the medical staff bylaws. When a precautionary suspension lasts for more than 14 days or in the event an receives notice of a recommendation by the MEC that will adversely affect his or her exercise of clinical privileges, the APP and his or her supervising physician shall have the right to meet personally with [two physicians and a peer] assigned by the president of the medical staff to discuss the recommendation. The APP and the supervising physician must request such a meeting in writing to the CEO within 30 working days from the date of receipt of such notice. At the meeting, the APP and the supervising physician must be present to discuss, explain, or refute the recommendation, but such meeting shall not constitute a hearing as noted in the medical staff bylaws for medical staff members, and none of the procedural rules set forth in the medical staff bylaws with respect to hearings shall apply. Findings from this review body will be forwarded to the affected practitioner, the MEC, and the board.

The APP and the supervising physician may request an appeal in writing to the CEO within [X] days of receipt of the findings of the review body. [Two members of the board assigned by the chair of the board or MEC] shall hear the appeal from the APP and the supervising physician. A representative from medical staff leadership may be present. The decision of the appeal body will be forwarded to the board for final decision. The APP and the supervising physician will be notified within [X] days of the final decision of the board.

  

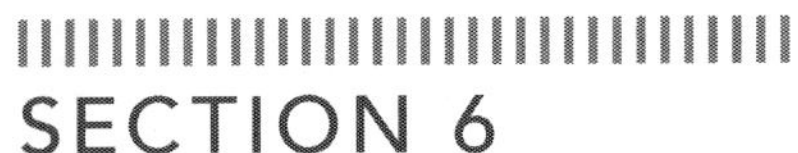

SECTION 6

# Medical Staff Operational Issues

Medical staffs today are, more than ever before, challenged by the time constraints of their members. More administrative physicians (i.e., chief medical officer, vice president of medical affairs, administrative medical director, etc.) are taking on roles that alleviate some of the time burden on medical staff leaders, whose primary responsibility is the care of their own patients. Moreover, more medical staffs are redesigning their medical staff operations to alleviate some of the burden placed on their members by, for example, centralizing certain medical staff functions and streamlining the medical staff committee structure and process.

## Streamlining the Medical Staff Committee Structure and Process

Medical staff documents must address the many administrative issues that are required to facilitate the smooth operation of the organization. When redesigning your medical staff structure, consider the number of committees and meeting attendance and quorum requirements. Are they all necessary to the operations of the medical staff?

This section covers some of the infrastructure requirements and functions that accrediting agencies and the Centers for Medicare & Medicaid Services (CMS) insist medical staffs address.

### *Medical staff functions*

CMS and accrediting agencies enumerate myriad functions that medical staffs must address. One tactic to ensure that the medical staff addresses all of the required functions is to list them in a section of the medical staff documents. In the past, medical staffs often formed a committee to address each of the functions required by CMS, but given physicians' lack of time, medical staffs should rethink this strategy. Typically, such a list of required functions (and committees) is located in an organization and functions manual.

The organization and functions manual is also a road map for identifying which individual(s) or committee(s) is accountable for specific medical staff responsibilities. The medical staff officers, department chairs, and medical staff or hospital committees are responsible for communicating regularly with the medical executive committee (MEC) so that it can ensure adherence to regulatory and accreditation standards. The ultimate responsibility for all medical staff functions lies with the MEC.

When creating language describing the functions of individuals and committees, it is useful to simply recite the functional responsibilities exactly as listed in CMS and various accreditation agency medical staff standards. You don't want to create overly grand bylaws that you are unable to comply with. You will be held accountable to the higher standard you create.

If the MEC creates a committee that is responsible for medical care evaluation, performance improvement, and patient safety activities, CMS requires that committee to:

- Perform competency assessment (e.g., ongoing professional practice evaluation [OPPE], if the hospital is Joint Commission–accredited)
- Recommend focused review of practitioners (such as focused professional practice evaluation [FPPE] per The Joint Commission [TJC]) when concerns arise from OPPE based on the general competencies defined by the medical staff
- Set expectations and define individual and aggregate measures to assess current clinical competency, provide feedback to practitioners, and develop plans for improving the quality of clinical care provided
- Be involved in the measurement, assessment, and improvement of practitioner performance that include, but are not limited to, evaluating a practitioner's:
  - Medical assessment and treatment of patients
  - Use of medications
  - Use of blood and blood components
  - Operative and other procedures
  - Education of patients and families
  - Accurate, timely, and legible completion of patients' medical records to include the quality of medical histories and physical examinations

  

  - Appropriateness of clinical practice patterns
  - Significant departures from established pattern of clinical performance
  - Use of developed criteria for autopsies
  - Sentinel event data
  - Patient safety data
  - Coordination of care, treatment, and services with other practitioners and hospital personnel, as relevant to the care, treatment, and services of an individual patient
  - Findings of the assessment process relevant to individual performance
- Communicate findings, conclusions, recommendations, and actions to improve the performance of practitioners to medical staff leaders and the board, and define in writing who is responsible for following up with the practitioner improvement plan

The medical staff should also participate in hospital performance improvement and patient safety programs to:

- Understand the medical staff's and administration's approach to and methods of performance improvement
- Assist the hospital to ensure that important processes and activities to improve performance and patient safety are measured, assessed, and spread systematically across all disciplines
- Identify and manage sentinel events and events that warrant intensive analysis (as requested)
- Measure, analyze, and manage variation in the processes that affect patient care to help reduce medical errors (as requested)
- Determine the appropriate number of medical staff committees

SAMPLE BYLAWS LANGUAGE

### Responsibilities of the medical staff

The organized medical staff is actively involved in the measurement, assessment, and improvement of the functions outlined in Section [X], and the ultimate responsibility lies with the MEC. The medical staff officers, department chairs, and hospital and medical staff committee chairs are responsible for working collaboratively to accomplish required medical staff functions. This process may include periodic reports as appropriate to the department/committee. It may also include elevating certain issues to the MEC as needed to ensure adherence to regulatory/accreditation compliance and appropriate standards of medical care.

## Determining the Appropriate Number of Medical Staff Committees

Why do some medical staffs have up to 20 standing committees? Simply put, some medical staffs rush to create a new committee every time an accreditation agency publishes another function that requires medical staff participation.

Originally, the MEC performed all of the functions required by the medical staff. However, as requirements and mandated functions grew, the MEC began to establish standing subcommittees to accomplish various tasks. If a streamlined infrastructure is the goal, a medical staff with a strong MEC, credentials committee, and multi-specialty quality/peer review committee can carry out almost all the work of the medical staff.

Various accreditation standards, regulations, laws, and professional organizations (e.g., medical societies) may require the establishment of some committees. For example, the American College of Surgeons mandates a trauma committee if the facility wants to be certified as a trauma center. Many of these committees can be designated as hospital committees with medical staff participation (discussed later in this section). Although these are the most commonly required committees, keep in mind that some state laws may require additional committees (e.g., safety committee and pharmacy committee). All other committees are optional, and you should consider keeping them only if they provide value to the organization. Each medical staff must decide for itself whether a committee provides value.

## Medical Staff Versus Hospital Committees

Many committees that have historically been organized under the medical staff might function just as well (or better) as a multidisciplinary hospital committee with designated physician participation. The president of the medical staff can appoint designated physician leaders to serve on hospital committees to help fulfill medical staff functions. This seems to work well for committees that address blood usage, utilization review, medical records, ethics, pharmacy/therapeutics, and infection control.

For example, a medical staff ethics committee could become a hospital committee with physician representation. Under this structure, the MEC would no longer be directly accountable for that committee's functions, but physician representatives on the committee would keep the MEC abreast of important issues. Although the medical staff must play a role in a wide variety of hospital functions—such as blood-usage monitoring, participation in ethical decision-making, selecting formulary drugs, and adopting infection control policies—it need not manage a long list of committees to serve those purposes. Another alternative to medical staff or hospital committees is to enlist the services of designated physician liaisons, advisors, or experts.

For example, the medical staff could replace a long-standing medical staff infection control committee with a physician advisor who meets regularly with the hospital infection control coordinator to address appropriate issues. This individual would report periodically and as necessary to the MEC (or medical staff quality committee), eliminating the need for a group of physicians to take the time to attend regular committee meetings. Consider addressing functions such as blood-usage monitoring or utilization review in this way as well.

  

Other medical staff committees need not be standing committees. Instead, they could function on an ad hoc basis. A bylaws committee might be called into existence whenever there is a perceived need to review or modify the medical staff governing documents. A physician advocacy/impaired physician committee could meet only as needed when a matter of physician health, well-being, or impairment arises. A joint conference committee of the medical staff and board might meet on an ad hoc basis only when there are differences of opinion between the MEC and the board or when requested by either party.

Traditionally, medical staffs appointed a nominating committee that convened on an ad hoc basis to develop a ballot prior to electing medical staff officers. Because the task of finding, educating, training, and retaining excellent medical staff leaders is becoming increasingly important, some medical staffs are now establishing an ongoing leadership and succession committee. This committee develops selection criteria, outlines a leadership training process, and works to create a pool of future leaders. This is one of the few committees that medical staffs should not eliminate in an effort to streamline medical staff operations.

Sometimes the medical staff resists having traditional medical staff committees become hospital committees with medical staff participation because they feel that the hospital will run roughshod over the medical staff. To prevent this from happening, there needs to be checks and balances in place such that when a hospital committee proposes actions that affect the clinical practice of privileged practitioners, those actions must be approved by the MEC before they can be enacted.

The MEC is ultimately accountable for all medical staff work and for ensuring that all medical staff functions are achieved. It can accomplish its work through whatever committee infrastructure it deems most efficient. Given the extreme demands on physicians' time and the difficulty many medical staffs encounter trying to get physicians to attend meetings, less may be more when it comes to establishing a committee infrastructure.

There is one caveat to keep in mind if you plan to modify or simplify your medical staff's committees: Some states limit peer review protections to activities carried out by peer review committees. Check the wording of your state's statute to see if your bylaws must accommodate particular language to take advantage of these protections.

In addition to describing the number and primary functions of the standing committees of the medical staff, governing documents should address the following:

- How each committee's members are selected (appointment or election)
- Which individuals will chair each committee
- The terms of appointment
- The body to which each committee is accountable
- The key responsibilities of each committee

## Attendance and Quorum

The original set of model bylaws that TJC released in the late 1960s contained a requirement that medical staff members must attend a certain percentage of meetings. Although that requirement has long since been removed, many organizations' bylaws still contain language requiring members to attend a certain percentage of medical staff/department meetings. Some medical staffs now state that a member must attend a certain percentage of meetings to be eligible to vote the next year; others require physicians to attend major decision-making medical staff committee meetings, including the MEC, the credentials committee, and the medical staff quality/peer review committee.

Although TJC no longer requires medical staff members to attend a certain percentage of meetings, The Healthcare Facilities Accreditation Program (HFAP) still states that active staff members are expected to attend staff, department, and committee meetings. If your organization is HFAP–accredited, it must maintain attendance and quorum language in the medical staff bylaws.

  

If a medical staff has meeting attendance requirements that work, it should keep them. However, physicians' clinical practice today is vastly different from the way it was decades ago. Many physicians spend more time in the office and less time in the hospital. To keep their practices financially viable, they see more patients than ever before. Physicians have little time to attend meetings and, therefore, attendance at medical staff meetings is typically poor.

Medical staffs that try to enforce attendance requirements usually find it a frustrating endeavor. Few are willing to remove a physician from the staff for failing to meet medical staff meeting requirements. Although TJC does not require meeting attendance, it does hold medical staffs responsible for enforcing any requirements it places in its bylaws. Therefore, some medical staffs have revised their bylaws to minimize attendance requirements, even while medical staff leaders continue to seek ways to encourage participation in meetings. Most medical staffs acknowledge that they cannot mandate attendance, especially if the physicians don't find the meetings useful.

Nothing frustrates physicians more than being present at a meeting but not being able to conduct business because a quorum doesn't exist. Many staffs no longer require a quorum at general staff, department, or committee meetings. Their bylaws indicate that a quorum will be defined as "those present." Some create a quorum threshold of only three members to conduct business. These medical staffs are not worried that the few individuals present will implement some outlandish decision because they realize there are checks and balances in place. Usually, voting is limited to only those items on the agenda, which is distributed to all potential meeting attendees. Therefore, issues cannot be voted on without notice. If physicians are interested in the decision being made, they need to be there for the vote. Decisions affecting the entire medical staff must be forwarded to the MEC before they are passed. For the major decision-making medical staff committees (e.g., MEC, the credentials committee, and the medical staff quality/peer review committee), quorum requirements are usually maintained.

  

SAMPLE BYLAWS LANGUAGE

**Attendance requirements**

Members of the medical staff are encouraged to attend meetings of the medical staff. Members of the MEC, credentials committee, and medical staff quality/peer review committee are expected to attend at least [75%] of the meetings held [annually or over the term of the appointment].

SAMPLE BYLAWS LANGUAGE

**Required quorums for various committees**

Medical staff meetings: those voting members present

MEC, credentials committee, and medical staff quality/peer review committee: [50%] of voting members

Department meetings or medical staff committees other than those listed previously: those voting members present

## Confidentiality, Immunity, and Releases

Today's environment is more privacy- and security-conscious than ever. Whether it is in regard to a patient's medical information or the credentialing/peer review information of a practitioner, confidentiality must be addressed in the medical staff bylaws. This section addresses not only confidentiality issues, but also the immunity provisions provided to practitioners when performing their designated medical staff duties.

The medical staff bylaws or associated documents should clearly articulate the responsibilities for maintaining confidentiality when appropriate. Given some recent litigations, medical staff members need to fully understand their obligations to protect sensitive information and their immunities for engaging responsibly in medical staff activities.

## SAMPLE BYLAWS LANGUAGE

### Confidentiality, immunity, and releases

**Confidentiality of information:** To the fullest extent permitted by law, the following shall be kept confidential:

- Information submitted, collected, or prepared by any representative of this or any other healthcare facility, organization, or medical staff for the purposes of assessing, reviewing, evaluating, monitoring, or improving the quality and efficiency of healthcare provided
- Evaluations of current clinical competence and qualifications for staff appointment, affiliation, and/or clinical privileges or specified services
- Contributions to teaching or clinical research
- Determinations that healthcare services were indicated or performed in compliance with an applicable standard of care

This information will not be disseminated to anyone other than a representative of the hospital or to other healthcare facilities or organizations of health professionals that are engaged in official, authorized activities for which the information is needed. Such confidentiality shall also extend to information provided by third parties. Each practitioner expressly acknowledges that violations of confidentiality provided here are grounds for immediate and permanent revocation of staff appointment/affiliation and/or clinical privileges.

**Immunity from liability:** No representative of this healthcare organization shall be liable to a practitioner for damages or other relief for any decision, opinion, action, statement, or recommendation made within the scope of his or her duties as an official representative of the hospital or medical staff. No representative of this healthcare organization shall be liable for providing information, opinion, counsel, or services to a representative or to any healthcare facility or organization of health professionals concerning said practitioner. The immunity protections afforded in these bylaws are in addition to those prescribed by applicable state and federal law.

  

SAMPLE BYLAWS LANGUAGE

## Confidentiality, immunity, and releases (cont.)

**Covered activities:** The confidentiality and immunity provided by this article apply to all information or disclosures performed or made in connection with this or any other healthcare facility's or organization's activities concerning, but not limited to the following:

- Applications for appointment/affiliation, clinical privileges, or specified services
- Periodic reappraisals for renewed appointments/affiliations, clinical privileges, or specified services
- Corrective or disciplinary actions
- Hearings and appellate reviews
- Quality assessment and performance improvement/peer review activities
- Utilization review and improvement activities
- Claims reviews
- Risk management and liability prevention activities
- Other hospital, committee, department, or staff activities related to monitoring and maintaining quality and efficient patient care and appropriate professional conduct

**Release of information:** When requested by the president of the medical staff or designee, each practitioner shall execute general and specific releases. Failure to execute such releases shall result in an application for appointment, reappointment, or clinical privileges being deemed voluntarily withdrawn and not processed further.

  

## Parliamentary Procedure

Medical staffs often refer to *Robert's Rules of Order* (a book on parliamentary procedure found at *www.robertsrules.com*) or similar texts in their bylaws to govern the conduct of meetings and medical staff procedures. However, in the experience of many, such references are ill-advised for several reasons. First, medical staffs are not parliaments and rarely need to follow parliamentary procedure. Second, it is highly unlikely that any medical staff member is an expert in *Robert's Rules of Order*, rendering calls for its use in meetings disruptive and confusing. Third, it is not uncommon to find someone who wishes to disrupt a meeting claiming to be knowledgeable about *Robert's Rules of Order*, while no one else is in a position to verify or disapprove the assertion on the spot. Medical staff leaders should be trained in meeting management to run the various medical staff meetings in a manner that facilitates achieving the medical staff's objectives. *Robert's Rules of Order* can be reserved for exceptional circumstances that call for a more regimented procedure.

### SAMPLE BYLAWS LANGUAGE

#### Parliamentary procedure

Medical staff and committee meetings shall be run in a manner determined by the chair of the meeting. When parliamentary procedure is needed, as determined by the chair or evidenced by a majority vote of those attending the meeting, the latest edition of *Robert's Rules of Order* shall determine procedure.

  

# A Guide to Bylaws Document Review

To conduct an effective review of your medical staff bylaws, you must first understand the controversies and dangers associated with such documents. Medical staff bylaws are becoming a subject of intense scrutiny due to two trends. The first is the escalating strain on physician-hospital relationships as these two parties increasingly compete with one another for revenue; the second is the rapid growth of corporate negligence lawsuits brought against hospitals.

With regard to the first trend, some healthcare industry insiders call this the era of "co-opetition," because physicians' relationships with hospitals are characterized by cooperation and competition. Unfortunately, medical staff bylaws have been used as a weapon in this struggle. On one hand, some physician groups hope to provide physicians with leverage against hospitals by using the bylaws to ward off change. On the other hand, some hospitals hope to use the bylaws to create conditions or obligations that better align physicians' and hospitals' interests.

Accreditation agencies have long held that bylaws must be the product of mutual agreement between the hospital governing board and its medical staff. In other words, neither party can unilaterally amend the bylaws and still remain in compliance with accreditation standards. However, this has not stopped parties from arguing about what should be in the bylaws and debating over the process for amending and adopting bylaws.

## Economic Credentialing

Economic credentialing refers to the practice of placing emphasis not only on the quality of medical care that practitioners provide, but also on economic issues, such as their ability to rein in costs or on whether they are in competition with the organization as an owner of a competing facility. Three decades ago, no one would have imagined that utility and efficiency considerations could become part of the credentialing process. Even two decades ago, the notion that a physician's entrepreneurialism could lead the medical staff to disqualify him or her was virtually unheard of. Yet economic credentialing is quickly becoming part of mainstream practice in more hospitals. Many boards are reluctant to approve bylaws provisions that might limit their ability to create conflict-of-interest criteria for medical staff membership.

However, physician groups, including the AMA and some state medical societies, have rallied against bylaws provisions, referring to conflict-of-interest statements placed in medical staff bylaws as economic credentialing.

Economic credentialing also stems from the new focus on the fiduciary and fiscal responsibilities that have been placed on hospital boards in today's post-Enron business climate. Boards are under increased pressure to take control of and responsibility for the conduct of their hospitals' affairs. This imperative for greater control brings boards into conflict with the traditional model of hospital governance, under which the medical staff directs and controls the provision of care.

For that reason, the concept of economic credentialing touches a raw nerve for some physicians. It has come to symbolize the loss of autonomy and the loss of the luxury of practicing medicine without constant regard for the bottom line.

With that in mind, it is easy to understand why physician groups have sought to inject barriers into medical staff bylaws that limit the discretion of hospitals to restrict medical staff membership. This struggle is often intensified in states where courts have interpreted the medical staff bylaws as a contract between physicians and the hospital.

When the bylaws are considered a contract, physicians can use breach-of-contract arguments to seek injunctions against hospitals that deviate from their bylaws. Technically, both parties can seek contractual remedies if the bylaws are breached.

## Liability Risk Created by Bylaws

As previously stated, one of the trends involving bylaws is the rapid growth of corporate negligence lawsuits brought against hospitals. Because bylaws exist to describe how the medical staff carries out its responsibilities, plaintiffs who are suing hospitals often claim that any deviation in practice from those detailed in the bylaws is by nature a negligent practice.

Historically, a lawsuit that alleged medical malpractice was directed at the physician(s) providing the patient's care. Today, plaintiffs' attorneys frequently attempt to add the medical staff and hospital as defendants by alleging that there was a failure to meet the bylaws' standards for credentialing and monitoring the physician(s) who provided care.

The argument goes as follows: If the hospital had not granted privileges to the physician against whom the malpractice claim was filed, the patient would not have been harmed. Following the same reasoning, if the hospital had adequately monitored the quality of the physician's performance, any substandard performance would have been detected before a patient (the plaintiff in the lawsuit) was injured. In addition, plaintiffs' attorneys often scrutinize the medical staff bylaws to determine whether the hospital followed the credentialing and peer review procedures outlined in these governing documents.

Attorneys use ambiguous or confusing bylaws language to argue that the hospital and medical staff were negligent and noncompliant. Further, when the processes described in a hospital's bylaws are overly complex or burdensome, attorneys claim there is an increased risk that medical staff leaders will deviate from strict bylaws compliance. If the medical staff fails to meticulously observe the details in the bylaws, plaintiffs' attorneys have yet another chance to claim negligence.

In some lawsuits, the plaintiffs are not patients, but rather physicians who believe that the medical staff has treated them improperly by restricting their privileges or terminating their medical staff membership. In such suits, the due-process provisions of the medical staff become the subject of intense scrutiny.

Poorly written bylaws can make such lawsuits more likely and even put at risk the legal immunities for peer review on which medical staffs rely. When the bylaws contain complicated or onerous due process provisions, medical staff members are less likely to comply with them meticulously; such lapses have cost hospitals millions of dollars in judgments.

## Undertaking a Bylaws Review

The importance of medical staff bylaws should compel every hospital and its medical staff leaders to ensure that bylaws are adequate, accurate, and in compliance with applicable requirements. A thorough review of these documents should occur periodically to determine whether they:

- Accurately reflect the structures and processes used by the medical staff
- Incorporate recognized leading practices for medical staff functioning and structure
- Are organized into a user-friendly and flexible set of documents
- Adequately address potential future conflicts
- Comply with regulatory standards

  

Keep in mind that your organization should assess the bylaws on an annual basis and whenever a regulatory body introduces a new standard or makes changes to an existing standard. However, a thorough assessment of your bylaws can occur less frequently.

For example, some medical staffs automatically conduct a comprehensive bylaws document review every three to five years. Others undertake this task only when they decide it is necessary to take a rigorous look at, and possibly redesign, the medical staff structure and processes to ensure that they perform efficiently and effectively. This type of medical staff redesign would provide a great opportunity to review these documents.

Do not allow more than three to five years between thorough bylaws assessments. Unfortunately, too many medical staff bylaws documents resemble archaeological finds. Every year the number of pages in the document grows as essential new additions are layered on top of old and often unnecessary provisions. Many times, a casual read-through of the bylaws results in the identification of medical staff "fixes" that were inserted to address a problem that last surfaced more than 10 years ago.

The result is an unwieldy and ossified document that hinders the effectiveness of a modern medical staff in a rapidly evolving healthcare environment. If this describes your bylaws, it may be time to consider a comprehensive review and potential top-to-bottom overhaul.

## Responsibility for the Bylaws Review

A designated MSP should keep the medical executive committee (MEC) up to date on regulations and standard changes that might affect the bylaws.

Some medical staffs have a standing bylaws committee. Suggestions for appropriate bylaws revisions can be vetted through this group or through an alternate medical staff process. However, the medical staff leadership (with the endorsement of the MEC) can and should make the decision to undertake a thorough review of the medical staff's governing documents. Keep in mind that this activity will inevitably be tinged with organizational politics and should be carefully planned.

Standing bylaws committee members may have a vested interest in the old documents. In some organizations, the chair of the bylaws committee has held the position for many years and therefore may have an ownership mentality regarding the current bylaws and may resist significant changes to the documents.

The MEC may want to consider appointing a special task force to undertake the review. Appointees can be chosen for their knowledge of medical staff affairs, ability to craft good bylaws language, ability to influence medical staff members to accept the changes, statesmanship, and other critical qualities.

When redesigning the bylaws (and redesigning the medical staff), these are the areas that usually need to be addressed:

- Membership
  - What types of practitioners qualify for membership
  - Membership responsibilities
  - Membership rights
- Leadership
  - Determination of which medical staff officer positions are necessary for a smoothly functioning medical staff
  - Qualifications of leaders
  - Election and removal processes
- Department
  - The necessary number of departments
  - Which medical staff members qualify to be department chairs
- Committees

  

  - Medical staff versus hospital committees
  - MEC/credentials/medical staff quality
  - Composition of committees
  - Functions of committees
- Meetings
  - Attendance
  - Quorum
  - Voting

## Enable the Creation of New Bylaws

Careful vetting of current bylaws and thoughtful rewriting or reorganizing are only the first steps along the path to developing new medical staff governing documents. The next challenge is overcoming resistance to change. Remember, resistance to change is universal and typically greatest in volatile times such as those we now face in healthcare.

Once a committee or task force recommends change, it should create and fully explain the new draft document to medical staff leadership. The "buy-in" of medical staff leaders is essential, and every effort should be made to achieve consensus at this level. The committee or task force should then plan a campaign to educate and win the acceptance of the general medical staff.

Common tools in the effort to educate the medical staff are town-hall meetings, newsletters, presentations by leadership at department meetings, and one-on-one meetings with physicians who are most likely to resist change. The eventual goal, of course, is to win the acceptance necessary to ensure that the bylaws can be modified under the amendment procedure in the current bylaws.

## Conclusion

The 21st century demands that practitioners change the way they deliver healthcare to patients. Hospitals are likely to continue their rapid pace of change, and the nature of the organized medical staff must change as well. If your medical staff bylaws are a hindrance to innovative change, you may hobble your institution and its practitioners. I hope that the guidance provided in this book will facilitate the evolution of medical staffs into highly effective and efficient organizations.

In my consulting work with medical staffs, I have always been impressed to see that revising bylaws is much more of a change management challenge than a clerical and scribing chore. When striving to achieve effective bylaws, we are well advised to keep in mind the wisdom of Albert Einstein: "Any intelligent fool can make things bigger, more complex . . . It takes a touch of genius—and a lot of courage—to move in the opposite direction."

As was noted in the Introduction, it was also Einstein who admonished us that "All things should be made as simple as possible, but not more so." These are words to live by for all of us who endeavor to improve medical staff bylaws.

  